Staying Dry:
A Practical Guide to Bladder Control

Staying Dry

A Practical Guide to Bladder Control

Dry

Kathryn L. Burgio, PH.D.
K. Lynette Pearce, R.N., C.R.N.P.
Angelo J. Lucco, M.D.

The Johns Hopkins University Press
Baltimore and London

The Johns Hopkins University Press,
701 West 40th Street,
Baltimore, Maryland 21211
The Johns Hopkins Press Ltd., London

The paper used in this publication meets the minimum
requirements of American National Standard for Information
Sciences—Permanence of Paper for Printed Library
Materials, ANSI Z39.48-1984.

Library of Congress Cataloging-in-Publication Data

Burgio, Kathryn.
    Staying dry : a practical guide to bladder control /
  Kathryn L. Burgio, K. Lynette Pearce, Angelo J. Lucco.
        p.   cm.
    Includes index.
    ISBN 0-8018-3912-2.—ISBN 0-8018-3909-2 (pbk.)
    1. Urinary incontinence—Popular works.   I. Pearce,
  K. Lynette, 1946–   .   II. Lucco, Angelo J., 1951–   .
  III. Title.
  RC921.I5B87   1989
  616.8′49—dc20   89-45480
                                                 CIP

To our mothers—
Maureen, Dorothy, and Ruth
—with love

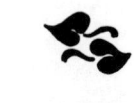

Contents

viii   Contents

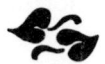

Foreword

In the past few years, millions of Americans have become zealous believers in self-help for good health. A half-hour in a good bookstore will expose you to a colorful array of hard- and softbound volumes dedicated to decreasing stress, cholesterol, blood sugar, and your waistline, and more volumes directed at increasing energy, personal effectiveness, sexual pleasure, and your children's potty skills or IQ scores. Dozens of additional books do not offer remedies for health conditions but describe and discuss a particular disease or health problem in great detail and present all the facts of the condition in simple language.

Conspicuous by its absence has been a book that explains a very common condition called incontinence. Incontinence, simply defined, is the inability to go to the bathroom when you want to and where you want to. An estimated ten million Americans are affected to some degree by urinary incontinence. Infection, inflammation, loss of female hormones after the menopause in women, obesity, prostate enlargement in men, diabetes—these are among the many factors that can cause changes in bladder function. There are numerous treatments and combinations of therapies to restore or improve bladder control—from weight reduction and hormone replacement to pelvic floor muscle exercises and surgery. But people will not benefit from any of these successful treatments until they (1) admit they have the condition; (2) explore the cause and nature of their problem; and (3) participate in their care to the best of their ability. Until now, these requirements have been made difficult by a shameful lack of information. People have kept their "secret." It is estimated that only one in twelve adults tells a doctor—or anyone else for that matter—about this embarrassing symptom.

We know from research done by our organization that many people believe they are incontinent because they are aging. This is simply not true. It is true that some age-related conditions cause people to have changes in bladder habits and control. Many of these changes can be handled with information provided in this book. We know also from our research that people haven't known where to go or what to do to begin helping themselves once they do admit to a problem. Now they have all the answers—right here in this book.

When Help for Incontinent People (HIP) was founded in 1982, it was designed to fill the void of silence and despair about incontinence with information and understanding about successful treatments and management options. As successful as we have been, we know we have reached only a few hundred thousand out of the millions of people who are affected. In 1984, our National Agenda to Promote Urinary Continence cited the desperate need for information for the lay public. In 1988, the National Institutes of Health sponsored a Consensus Development Conference on Urinary Incontinence in Adults. Again, the importance of public education was emphasized. This valuable book is right on target. It presents the subject in simple and tasteful style, explains very complicated tests and procedures in understandable language, and offers safe and reasonable solutions for many people. It does not interfere with the doctor-patient relationship or minimize the importance of the doctor in the diagnosis and treatment of bladder control problems. It is a timely and welcome addition to the health and self-help section of American bookstores and libraries.

Many readers will be comforted simply by the knowledge that they are not the only ones who suffer from this condition. Many more will be delighted to know that there are exercises that they can do in the privacy of their home that are safe and effective. Others will be pleased to find that they can actively participate in their care and assist their doctor in finding the cause and the proper treatment for their condition. This book blends the unique talents and experiences of a behavioral psychologist, a nurse, and a physician. This book, in a word, is wonderful. Read on.

Katherine F. Jeter, Ed.D., E.T., Director
Help for Incontinent People, Inc.
Union, South Carolina 29379

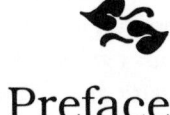

Preface

During the course of our research at the National Institute on Aging, we spent many hours working with older women and men who had problems with bladder control. We listened as they spoke of the embarrassment they suffered with each accident and the distress of losing an ability once taken for granted. We saw their hopelessness and, at times, felt helpless ourselves. Then we watched, sometimes with surprise, always with pleasure, as these same people regained bladder control. We saw healthy, active people once isolated by this problem take charge of their lives. Impressed with their eagerness to learn about incontinence and the active role they took in their own health care, we realized the potential for many thousands of people to do the same and we began to write this book. Incontinence is hidden and it is ignored, but incontinence is not a hopeless problem. We thank these people who shared an uncomfortable part of their lives with us.

Along the way, we were encouraged by the interest and support of many colleagues and friends. We are especially grateful to Bernard T. Engel, Ph.D., Chief of the Laboratory of Behavioral Sciences, Gerontology Research Center, National Institute on Aging, who initiated and guided the program of research that stimulated our interest in incontinence. Dr. Engel's groundbreaking research on the treatment of incontinence set the stage for our own work in this area. His support, suggestions, and critical feedback during our research and the development of this book were invaluable.

We thank William E. Whitehead, Ph.D., of the Johns Hopkins University School of Medicine, who taught us many of the basic principles and techniques that appear in this book. In addition, he developed the original bladder record which is the prototype for our bladder diary.

We appreciate the ongoing support of John R. Burton, M.D., of the Johns Hopkins University School of Medicine, who initiated the incontinence research project that brought us together.

We are grateful to Diane A. Jakovac Smith, R.N., M.S.N., C.R.N.P., a nurse practitioner and colleague from Golden Horizons, Inc., Newtown Square, Pennsylvania, who worked with us in the development of our ideas for the book in its early stages.

We also wish to thank the following trusted colleagues, friends, and relatives who took time out of their busy schedules to read various drafts of this book and, by sharing their constructive criticism, helped to make it an accurate and useful guide.

• Carol A. Brink, M.P.H., R.N., University of Rochester School of Nursing

• Louis D. Burgio, Ph.D., University of Pittsburgh School of Medicine

• Dorothy Candib, M.D., University of Pittsburgh School of Medicine

• Susan J. Denman, M.D., The Johns Hopkins University School of Medicine

- Bernard T. Engel, Ph.D., Gerontology Research Center, National Institute on Aging
- J. Andrew Fantl, M.D., Medical College of Virginia, Virginia Commonwealth University
- Cheryle B. Gartley, The Simon Foundation
- Katherine F. Jeter, Ed.D., E.T., Help for Incontinent People
- B. Joan McDowell, Ph.D., C.R.N.P., University of Pittsburgh School of Medicine
- Harvey N. Schonwald, M.D., Urologist, Baltimore, Maryland
- Ray E. Stutzman, M.D., The Johns Hopkins University School of Medicine
- Jean F. Wyman, Ph.D., R.N.C., School of Nursing, Virginia Commonwealth University/Medical College of Virginia
- Mary Gabryszewski Burgio, R.N., B.S.N., Buffalo, New York
- Pamela A. Burgio, R.N., B.S.N., United States Air Force Nurse Corps
- Angeline M. Godson, Buffalo, New York
- Jay Arthur Heck, J.D., Baltimore, Maryland
- Maureen C. Larsen, R.N., Northfield, Vermont
- Elizabeth M. Lipomi, Buffalo, New York

Joseph Flynn of We're Printing Today, Elizabeth, New Jersey, printed our bladder diary forms and exercise calendars. Gaddiel Lopez of Baltimore, Maryland, provided the initial illustrations and Elizabeth Sanders, also of Baltimore, designed the final illustrations. We appreciate their talent, as well as their patience during multiple revisions.

And we are indebted to the Johns Hopkins University Press, especially to science editor Wendy Harris, for guiding us through the process of turning our final manuscript into this final product. Most importantly, we commend them for fulfilling their goal of conveying medical information to the general public by publishing this book, while dozens of other publishers simply told us the topic was not "marketable."

We offer our sincere wish that you, our readers, will grasp the information presented and take action to improve your bladder control. We welcome comments that will make subsequent editions of this work more helpful to future readers.

Kathryn L. Burgio
K. Lynette Pearce
Angelo J. Lucco

Although many people encouraged our efforts to complete this book, I might never have finished my part were it not for the support and encouragement of my husband Lou. As my friend and my professional colleague, he respects my work as he respects his own, and as a "super dad" of the eighties, he proved it by taking care of a four-year-old and infant twins during my several absences to work on the book. I'm also grateful to my daughters Emily, Kalyn, and Jaime for their cheerful tolerance of my hours away from them. Finally, I thank my parents, Fred and Maureen Larsen, whose life has set an example of hard work and giving that has helped me to experience great satisfaction in putting forth a book written to help others.

KLB

I would like to thank my family, who have supported me always: my sister and brother-in-law, Dorothy and

Jack Clarke; my mother, Dorothy Pearce Schildt; and my stepfather, Ellis Schildt. They have stood close by, but just far enough away. As we publish this book, I think of my dad, Manley Pearce, and Ray Hasselhoff as I have thought of them at every milestone in my life—wishing that they could have stayed with me longer. And finally, my thanks to the man who kept my lawn mowed as I worked on the book, the best "neighbor" in the world—Bill Sewell.

KLP

Anjanette, Alissa, Danielle, Joe, Sharon, Sue, Fred, Jane, Frank, Marion, Pat, Dick; Jay; Dean, Sharlene, Michael, Steve, Herb, Ed, Ron, Dave, Linda, Sue; Ron, Frank, Michael; Lynette, Kathy; Ruth (see dedication) and my dad—he would have loved to see this.

AJL

INTRODUCTION

From Damp to Dry

Urinary incontinence is the accidental loss of urine—wetting yourself. It is an embarrassing and expensive problem that troubles millions of people, men and women, young and old. Yet, most people know very little about it or where to turn for help. This book is your guide.

This book is for every adult who suffers from urinary incontinence—whether you have never told anyone about your problem or whether you have discussed it with your doctor and yet still leak urine. This book explains the different types of incontinence as well as the various treatments available. You will learn a series of exercises and strategies that, when practiced carefully, can significantly improve or cure most types of incontinence.

You Are Not Alone

Loss of bladder control affects at least *one of every ten* adults. In its mildest form, incontinence is a mere annoyance. When it is severe, it becomes a disturbing condition that can lead to serious restrictions in your normal daily life. Consider Susan's story.

Susan's problem with bladder control started when she was fifty-two years old. At first, it was a minor problem that she easily controlled by wearing sanitary napkins. Gradually, however, it became worse. Eventually, she not only leaked urine when she coughed, sneezed, or got up from a chair, but she also had accidents when she had a strong urge to urinate and could not make it to the bathroom in time. She told no one, not even her doctor.

As a real estate agent, Susan spent many of her days with clients touring homes around Portland, walking up and down stairs and getting in and out of her car. She began to wear adult diapers to be certain that her leakage would not be detected by clients and co-workers. After every journey, her diaper was saturated with urine and she began to worry about odor. She feared that others would notice, so she retired and spent most of her time at home. In an attempt to avoid accidents by keeping her bladder empty, she drank less and went to the bathroom more often. When she did go out, she did not allow herself to drink and she was preoccupied with the location of the next bathroom that she would need. Outings became a serious burden, and she avoided leaving home for any reason, even for a family wedding. Still, she told no one.

Susan's husband suspected that she had a problem, but they never discussed it. Concerned about wetting and odor, Susan avoided sex, and much of the intimacy was lost from their twenty-seven–year marriage. Restricting her activities to those that required the least body movement, she gradually adopted an extremely sedentary and isolated life. She was living her entire life around her bladder. Still she told no one and suffered in silence.

Susan thought that she was alone. Nothing could have been farther from the truth.

How Many People Have Problems with Bladder Control?

More than ten million American adults suffer with incontinence. Incontinence is more common among women, especially women over age sixty. Half of all women experience incontinence at some point in their lives. About one-third develop a regular problem with bladder control. Men are less likely to develop incontinence; nevertheless, about one of every five older men has urinary incontinence.

If It's So Common, Why Don't We Hear about It?

Most people don't talk about it. In our culture, incontinence is an unacceptable problem. Those who have never had the problem, and even those who do, commonly see incontinence as "dirty." We freely accept that babies wet their diapers and children have problems with bladder control. But beyond age four or five, everyone is expected to have perfect bladder control. "Babies can't help it; adults can."

This attitude shows a lack of understanding. For entirely legitimate medical reasons, sometimes adults can't help it either. Incontinence is not a lack of will. It is not a weakness of character or a regression to childhood. It is not a disease. Like a fever or a limp, it is a symptom, a physical sign of an underlying disorder. Incontinence is a medical condition that should be treated with the same concern and respect as any other medical problem.

Nevertheless, because our society does not always recognize this fact, loss of bladder control becomes an embarrassment, something to hide. And most people go to great lengths to hide it. Here are some of the adjustments that we have seen people with bladder control problems make:

- drinking as little as possible
- going to the bathroom frequently
- avoiding travel
- not attending meetings or going to church
- not lifting anything
- not going shopping
- avoiding sports or physical activities
- wearing pads or diapers
- wearing only dark clothes

One woman stopped going on bus trips with her travel club because the bus didn't stop often enough for her to go to the bathroom and she was uncomfortable most of the time. One man declined to accept an award for service at his Kiwanis Club because he was afraid of having an accident on stage. One man skipped his daughter's wedding. One woman canceled the fiftieth wedding anniversary party her children had planned. One woman refused to accompany her husband on the European trip that they had planned for their first year of retirement. One man declined a nomination to run for state office. One woman never lifted her grandchildren for fear of having an accident.

These people made adjustments in their lives that led to significant losses. They lost many chances to share important moments with family and friends. Considering these losses, it is not surprising that many people with incontinence become withdrawn, depressed, or upset. Too many people feel alone with this problem, and too many suffer in silence.

What Can Be Done?

The last thing you should do is suffer in silence. Urinary incontinence is a treatable condition. *In most cases, incontinence can be greatly reduced or eliminated.*

Urinary incontinence has many treatments. There are behavioral training procedures, including the exercises and skills that will be presented later in this book. A number of medicines have been helpful for some types of incontinence. Sometimes surgery is the answer. There are many people who can help you, and, most important, there are many ways to help yourself. This book is your guide to all of these options.

Why Don't People Get Help?

Some people don't seek help for incontinence because they are not bothered by it. Most of them are women with mild forms of urine loss that do not interfere with their everyday lives. But you must understand the possible consequences of ignoring this problem: Your loss of bladder control could get better on its own, it could stay the same, or it could get worse.

No one can predict with certainty which will happen in your case if you ignore the problem. But we do see many people who come for help only after they are desperate. As they look back, they realize that their incontinence slowly grew worse over the course of many years. We are able to help most of these people, but it is usually easier to treat incontinence when it is mild. It seems sad that these people suffered through years of concealment, humiliation, and solitude that could have been avoided.

Facts about Incontinence

People who are genuinely troubled with incontinence face several barriers to treatment. Most of them are myths.

Myth #1: "I'm not incontinent."

Fact: The first barrier to treatment is the difficulty of admitting that you have the problem. Losing a few drops of urine every time you laugh is easy to ignore. Even when the problem grows worse, many people are so ashamed that they persuade themselves that it is getting better. It is difficult to admit incontinence to yourself and face it directly. Taking action to tell your doctor about incontinence also takes courage, and it may cause you to feel anxious and embarrassed. But hurdling these barriers may open the door to a whole new life for you.

Myth #2: "I just can't tell my doctor."

Fact: The second barrier to seeking help may be your own attitude toward incontinence. If you share society's belief that loss of bladder control is not acceptable for discussion, not even with your doctor, try this thought:

Incontinence is a medical condition, and it deserves the same attention as any other medical condition. I would go to the doctor if I lost my eyesight. I should go to the doctor for my lost bladder control.

Don't be embarrassed; your doctor wants to help you. You can expect your doctor to evaluate your problem and describe the treatments that are appropriate for you. If your physician is not experienced in the evaluation and treatment of urinary incontinence, you should ask to be referred to someone who does have this experience.

Myth #3: "Incontinence is a natural part of growing older."

Fact: Incontinence is not an inevitable part of growing older, nor is it natural. Unfortunately, many people believe that incontinence is caused by age and, therefore, is irreversible. It is true that incontinence is more common in older people. As we age, some physical changes in the body make us more likely to lose bladder control. But incontinence is *not* caused by age itself. Most older people are dry.

Myth #4: "I'm too old."

Fact: You are never too old to receive medical attention for incontinence. Our experience in treating older men and women is that the types of incontinence they have and their response to treatment are quite similar to those of our younger patients. Don't let the mere fact of "being old" hold you back. Old dogs learn new tricks all the time.

Myth #5: "Incontinence is a natural part of bearing children."

Fact: Pregnancy and childbirth take a toll on a woman's body. The months of extra weight in the pelvis and the stretching and possible tearing of tissues during delivery have been known to damage structures that help to support the bladder and maintain good control of urine. Having babies may contribute to incontinence, but it does not necessarily mean that you have to be incontinent.

Knowing that your mother had bladder problems after giving birth and that the same thing happened to your sister and grandmother may tempt you to conclude that incontinence is not only natural but also inevitable. In some families and groups of women, incontinence is so accepted that it becomes a laughing matter. Although laughter can be good medicine, be sure that you are not laughing through your tears. Don't let the fact that other mothers leak convince you that it is a necessary part of life for you. Many women who started leaking after childbirth are dry today.

Myth #6: "Incontinence is not treatable" or "My case is hopeless."

Fact: *In most cases, incontinence is treatable,* and significant improvement or cure can be expected. For a number of reasons, this fact may not be apparent.

For all of the reasons discussed earlier, incontinence is not a popular topic of conversation. Facts about the problem and available treatments are not common knowledge. Most people are unaware that help is available. Only recently has there been advertising of incontinence products on television. Although these ads increase public awareness of the problem, their emphasis is on products that help people to live with incontinence. Without announcements that encourage people to see their doctors, viewers may conclude mistakenly that the problem is not treatable and that they should focus their efforts on finding the most comfortable and absorbent pad or diaper and learn to live with it.

Let's Get Started!

This book was written so that fewer people will "learn to live with incontinence." Treatment is available, and we will help you find it. In five steps, we will help you to evaluate your own problem and understand why you have lost bladder control. We will prepare you for a visit to your doctor by describing the procedures used to evaluate this condition and the treatments that you may be offered.

Most important, we will teach you what you can do for yourself—tried and true methods that have helped thousands, like Susan, regain bladder control.

How to Use This Book

The program is presented in five steps. To achieve the best results, begin with Step One and complete the work in each step of the program before you move ahead. We have provided space for you—right in the book—to answer questions and to keep a diary of your problem and your experiences as you progress. This is not "busywork." All of the information that you collect will be used in your treatment program. Everything you need is in this book, except a sharp pencil and a sincere desire to help yourself.

We strongly advise you not to read the entire book before you begin working on your problem. Get involved right from the start because each step depends on the knowledge you gained and the information you collected in the previous steps. Begin with Step One and work through one step at a time.

Step One teaches you how to examine your problem by keeping a diary of your bladder habits.

Step Two helps you to understand what your bladder diary means. It also provides an overview of the different types and causes of incontinence and helps you discover what type of incontinence you have. Although this book is a guide to helping yourself, *it is not in-*

tended to replace your doctor. A medical evaluation is an important and necessary part of this program, and guidelines are provided for choosing the health care provider who will best meet your needs.

Step Three tells you how to prepare for your medical evaluation and what to expect during your visit. Additional tests that may be performed are described in Appendix A. A detailed discussion of the treatments you may be offered, along with the risks and benefits of each one, can be found in Appendix B.

Step Four teaches exercises that you can practice and skills that you can use, based on the type of incontinence you have, to achieve improved bladder control.

Step Five helps you to evaluate your progress and to make decisions about the need for further treatment.

The Glossary defines all of the important terms used in this book.

The Index allows you to find topics that you may want to read about a second time.

Staying Dry: A Practical Guide to Bladder Control is based on our years of experience helping people with various types of urinary incontinence. The program that we describe has helped thousands of men and women regain bladder control. If you read and follow the steps carefully, if you become involved and give it your best effort, we believe that you will achieve that same success. It all depends on you.

If you

- leak urine when you cough or sneeze

- have to run to the bathroom every fifteen minutes

- can't lift a grocery bag without leaking

- lose urine when you hear water running

- leak when you can't stop laughing

- know where every bathroom is at your local mall

- leak while standing on your doorstep with your keys in your hand

this book was written for you.

If your bladder controls your life, these five steps will put you back in charge. Turn the page and take control.

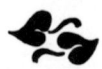

Getting a Handle on Your Problem

The first step in helping yourself is understanding your problem. A bladder diary will help you to do this. The diary will allow you to take a close look at the day-to-day picture of your urinary incontinence.

The importance of focusing on the problem by keeping a diary cannot be stressed enough. You must think of your diary as your constant companion. Your diary will not only provide a detailed picture of your problem, but will also be important in providing information for your doctor and in planning your treatment.

What Your Bladder Diary Will Tell You

Your diary will show you the exact number of accidents that you have each day. Many people underestimate the severity of their problem and are surprised at the number of accidents that they actually have. This experience is much like starting a diet and writing down everything you eat: usually we don't realize how much we are eating until we keep a written record.

Another important fact that you will learn by keeping a diary is what makes you leak, that is, what events and what movements cause you to lose urine. There may be times when leakage is caused by an obvious event, such as a sneeze. At other times, you may find yourself wet and not remember when or why you leaked. You may think that you know exactly what causes you to lose urine but will find, while keeping the diary, that there are other events of which you were not aware. Knowing precisely the events or movements that cause you to leak urine will be important later in planning your treatment. The strategies that you will learn to use to prevent leakage will help only if you know when to use them.

The diary will also make you more aware of other behaviors that you have acquired as a result of your problem. For example, you will notice how many times you go to the bathroom each day. Many people discover that they go to the bathroom every time they are near a toilet, even though, most of the time, they don't even have the urge to void (another word for urinate). Without knowing it, they formed this habit because they hoped to reduce incontinence by keeping their bladders empty. Unfortunately, frequent voiding can aggravate a problem with bladder control. For this reason, it is important to recognize bad bladder habits early.

Your diary will also help you to define the type of incontinence that you have. Knowing your type of incontinence is essential in planning your treatment program because different strategies are used for dealing with different types of incontinence.

Later, after you have completed the entire program, you will keep another diary. Then, you will go back to your first bladder diary to see how much you have improved.

How to Keep Your Bladder Diary

As your first step, keep a diary for one week. Remember that its main purpose is to look at what is normal for you. By keeping your diary, you are painting a picture of your problem. Go about your daily life and avoid making any changes in your bathroom habits.

Keeping your diary is essential and should not be taken lightly. It need not be fancy or neat, as long as it contains useful information. You should fill in your diary as the day goes by. Do not wait until the end of the day and then try to remember everything that happened. Write the information in your diary as you go along. It takes only seconds to do and is much more accurate if done right away.

The bladder diary is divided into four columns (see fig. 1). The column headings are: urinated in toilet, small accident, large accident, and reason for accident.

In the "urinated in toilet" column, you should record the exact time whenever you go to the bathroom.

The next two columns are "small accident" and "large accident." A small accident is a few drops of urine in your underpants or a moist pantyliner. A large accident is one that saturates a pad or wets your outer clothing. For each accident, record in the appropriate column the exact time that it occurred. Any leakage at all is considered an accident, even if it is just a few drops. If you are in doubt, count it as an accident.

Whenever you feel yourself leaking or find yourself damp, change your pad or clothing. This change will increase your awareness of when you are leaking and improve the accuracy of your diary. If you wear a pad and change it only when it is very wet, you will be unable to tell exactly how many leakages you are having. For instance, if you put on a dry pad at 8:00 a.m. and don't change it until 1:00 p.m., when it is very wet, there will be no way to tell how many leakages occurred during that period. Many people find that they are having more accidents than they thought.

The last column is "reason for accident." The comments written here may describe the feeling that accompanies leakage of urine, such as "felt a sudden need to void but just couldn't make it to the bathroom," "got an urge while running water and leaked urine on the way to the bathroom," or "had a desire to void for fifteen minutes but waited too long to go to the bathroom." If you have no urge to void before the accident, you should record any event or movement that may have caused the leakage. Some examples of these reasons are: "sneezed," "bending over," "laughed," or "doing aerobics." Each time you note an accident in the diary, you should also record the reason for it. At times, this may be difficult if you do not know what caused an accident. In this case, record what you were doing when the accident occurred, such as "watching T.V.," "reading," or "doing the dishes."

At the bottom of each page is a space for you to write any observations that you think might be important and may have an effect on your problem, such as "drank more coffee than usual today," "out shopping all day," "didn't have an urge to void but passed urine with a bowel movement," or "had a cold and coughed all day." You will want this information later, when you review your records with your doctor. (For now, ignore the line for total number of accidents in the lower right corner; that will be explained and filled in later during Step Two.)

Each diary page covers a twenty-four-hour period, starting with the first time you pass urine after midnight.

Remember, if you had an urge to void before the accident, write it down. If you had no urge but an event or movement may have caused the accident, write that down. If you had no urge and can identify no cause, write what you were doing when the accident occurred.

Sample Bladder Diary

date: _____

In the first column, write the time whenever you void in the toilet.
In the second and third columns, write the time whenever you have an
    accident.
For every accident, write the reason in the fourth column.

Urinated in toilet	Small accident	Large accident	Reason for accident

Comments: _____

_____

_____

Figure 1.   Total number of accidents today: _____

Let's Practice!

To give you a better idea of exactly how to make entries in your diary, we will walk through a day with a person who has a bladder control problem. The following is a list of activities over a twenty-four-hour period. Read through the events of the day and fill in the blank diary sheet as you go along (use fig. 2).

December 28

3:00 a.m.:   Urinated in the toilet.

5:00 a.m.:   Urinated in the toilet.

7:15 a.m.:   Awoke with a strong urge to void. Started to the bathroom but couldn't hold it. Urinated a large amount on the bathroom floor.

7:18 a.m.:   Finished urinating in the toilet.

8:30 a.m.:   Urinated in the toilet with a bowel movement.

10:00 a.m.:   Lifted a bag of groceries; leaked a few drops of urine in underwear. Changed underwear.

12:15 p.m.:   Urinated in the toilet.

12:30 p.m.:   Sneezed, leaked a few drops of urine, moistened pad. Changed pad.

4:00 p.m.:   Coming from the car to the house after going to the bank, made it to the front door. Put the key in the lock, got sudden urge to void, and had a large accident, wetting through underwear and slacks.

4:15 p.m.:   Urinated in the toilet.

6:00 p.m.:   Coughed, leaked urine, and wet pad. Changed pad.

8:00 p.m.:   Urinated in the toilet.

9:30 p.m.:   While sitting and watching T.V., wet pad without warning. Changed pad.

11:00 p.m.:   Urinated in the toilet.

ractice Bladder Diary

date: ——————

the first column, write the time whenever you void in the toilet.
the second and third columns, write the time whenever you have an
accident.
or every accident, write the reason in the fourth column.

Urinated in toilet	Small accident	Large accident	Reason for accident

mments: ———————————————————————
——————————————————————————
——————————————————————————

ure 2.

Total number of accidents today: ——————

Now check your record with the completed practice bladder diary (fig. 3).

Remember, for the purpose of your bladder diary, each day starts with the first time you pass urine after midnight.

And Now, for Real

Now that you've got the hang of it, it's time to get started on the real thing—*your* bladder diary!

You will find your first-week bladder diary on the pages that follow. Pick up your pencil and begin *now*. Date the pages and begin your diary. Carry this book with you and use it!

After you complete your first-week bladder diary, go on to Step Two.

Practice Bladder Diary Answers

date: _12/28_

In the first column, write the time whenever you void in the toilet.
In the second and third columns, write the time whenever you have an
    accident.
For every accident, write the reason in the fourth column.

Urinated in toilet	Small accident	Large accident	Reason for accident
3:00 am			
5:00 am			
		7:15 am	woke up - strong urge - couldn't hold.
7:18 am			
* 8:30 am			
	10:00 um		lifted bag of groceries
12:15 pm			
	12:30 pm		sneezed
		4:00 pm	came home - opening door had strong urge - couldn't hold
4:15 pm			
	6:00 pm		coughed
8:00 pm			
	9:30 pm		watching TV
11:00 pm			

Comments:

   * with bowel movement

Figure 3.

Total number of accidents today: ____6____

First-Week Bladder Diary   Day #1   date: _____

In the first column, write the time whenever you void in the toilet.
In the second and third columns, write the time whenever you have an
   accident.
For every accident, write the reason in the fourth column.

Urinated in toilet	Small accident	Large accident	Reason for accident

Comments:
_____

_____

_____

Total number of accidents today: _____

First-Week Bladder Diary   Day #2   date: _____

In the first column, write the time whenever you void in the toilet.
In the second and third columns, write the time whenever you have an accident.
For every accident, write the reason in the fourth column.

Urinated in toilet	Small accident	Large accident	Reason for accident

Comments: _____

_____

_____

Total number of accidents today: _____

First-Week Bladder Diary   Day #3   date: _____

In the first column, write the time whenever you void in the toilet.
In the second and third columns, write the time whenever you have an
    accident.
For every accident, write the reason in the fourth column.

Urinated in toilet	Small accident	Large accident	Reason for accident

Comments: _____

_____

_____

Total number of accidents today: _____

First-Week Bladder Diary   Day #4   date: _____

In the first column, write the time whenever you void in the toilet.
In the second and third columns, write the time whenever you have an
    accident.
For every accident, write the reason in the fourth column.

Urinated in toilet	Small accident	Large accident	Reason for accident

Comments: _____

_____

_____

Total number of accidents today: _____

First-Week Bladder Diary   Day #5   date: _____

In the first column, write the time whenever you void in the toilet.
In the second and third columns, write the time whenever you have an
  accident.
For every accident, write the reason in the fourth column.

Urinated in toilet	Small accident	Large accident	Reason for accident

Comments: _____

_____

_____

Total number of accidents today: _____

First-Week Bladder Diary   Day #6

In the first column, write the time whenever you void in the toilet.
In the second and third columns, write the time whenever you have an
accident.
For every accident, write the reason in the fourth column.

Urinated in toilet	Small accident	Large accident	Reason for accident

Comments:
_____
_____
_____

Total number of accidents today: _____

First-Week Bladder Diary   Day #7   date: _____

In the first column, write the time whenever you void in the toilet.
In the second and third columns, write the time whenever you have an
   accident.
For every accident, write the reason in the fourth column.

Urinated in toilet	Small accident	Large accident	Reason for accident

Comments: _____

_____

_____

Total number of accidents today: _____

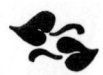

What Your First-Week Bladder Diary Means

Now that you have completed your first-week bladder diary, we will take a close look at it to see just what it means. The information from your bladder diary, along with your answers to the questions that follow, will provide you with a much clearer understanding of your problem. We call this a working diagnosis.

Based on your working diagnosis, we will begin planning your personal treatment program. You need to know what type of incontinence you have because different strategies are used for dealing with different types of incontinence. For the purpose of defining your problem, most incontinence is divided into two types: URGE incontinence and STRESS incontinence. Your answers to a few simple questions will provide information to help us classify the type of incontinence you have. Mark "yes" or "no" after each question.

Quick Quiz 1

	YES	NO
Do you have trouble making it to the toilet in time?	_____	_____
Do you lose urine when you have a strong urge to urinate?	_____	_____
Are you usually on the way to the bathroom when you lose urine?	_____	_____

	YES	NO

When you are coming home, can you usually make it to the door, but then lose urine just as you put the key in the lock?

Can you usually make it to the bathroom, but then lose urine just as you are getting to the toilet or removing your clothes?

While running water, do you sometimes get the urge to urinate and then are unable to make it to the toilet?

If you answered "yes" to any or all of these questions, your problem may be URGE incontinence. This means that your accidents occur when you experience a strong desire to void.

Quick Quiz 2

	YES	NO

Do you lose urine when you lift heavy objects, such as a basket of wet clothes or furniture?

Do you lose urine when you sneeze?

Do you lose urine when you bowl, run, or exercise?

Do you lose urine when you cough?

If you answered "yes" to any or all of these questions, your problem may be STRESS incontinence. This means that your accidents occur with activities that put pressure on your bladder.

After reading and answering both sets of questions, you may find that you answered "yes" to questions in both the URGE and STRESS categories. This means that you have both types of incontinence. This is known as MIXED incontinence and is very common.

Circle your working diagnosis here, based on your answers to the Quick Quizzes:

URGE   STRESS   MIXED

Reviewing Your First-Week Bladder Diary

Now, look closely at your first-week bladder diary. Let's go through the diary day by day and look at each time you wrote down an accident (small or large) and the reason for that accident. Start with your first accident on the first day. Does the accident seem related to having a strong urge to urinate, or does it seem to relate to a movement or event that caused increased pressure on your bladder? Another way to look at the accident is simply to ask, "Was the leakage at a time when you felt the urge to urinate or not?"

If you experienced the urge to void just before the accident, you should consider it an URGE-incontinent episode and place a "U" next to the accident on your diary sheet. Figure 4 is a sample diary page of someone who has a problem with URGE incontinence only. All of the accidents noted are related to having a strong urge to urinate. This person is generally on the way to the bathroom but is unable to get there before urine starts to flow.

If you did not experience an urge to void before the accident, ask yourself, "Could the leakage have been related to some form of movement or physical exertion?" If you can relate the accident to a physical movement, you should consider it a STRESS-incontinent episode and mark an "S" next to the accident on your diary sheet. Figure 5 is a sample diary page of someone

Sample Bladder Diary
Urge Incontinence

date: __1/8__

In the first column, write the time whenever you void in the toilet.

In the second and third columns, write the time whenever you have an accident.

For every accident, write the reason in the fourth column.

Urinated in toilet	Small accident	Large accident	Reason for accident
		ⓤ 5:55 am	*Strong urge – couldn't hold*
6:00 am			
9:10 am			
	ⓤ 10:30 am		*went out into the cold –*
			Strong urge – couldn't
			hold
12:00 pm			
2:10 pm			
		ⓤ 3:00 pm	*Strong urge – couldn't hold*
	ⓤ 5:20 pm		*urge – waited too long*
5:30 pm			
8:00 pm			
10:10 pm			

Comments:

Figure 4.

Total number of accidents today: __4__

Sample Bladder Diary
Stress Incontinence

date: _9/19_

In the first column, write the time whenever you void in the toilet.

In the second and third columns, write the time whenever you have an accident.

For every accident, write the reason in the fourth column.

Urinated in toilet	Small accident	Large accident	Reason for accident
7:10 am			
	(s) 7:30 am		doing sit-ups
9:00 am			
	(s) 10:10 am		lifted grocery bag
10:30 am			
	(s) 12:00 pm		sneezed
1:05 pm			
	(s) 2:30 pm		getting up from chair
5:00 pm			
	(s) 7:20 pm		laughing
9:00 pm			
	(s) 10:30 pm		coughing spell
11:45 pm			

Comments:

Figure 5.

Total number of accidents today: ___6___

who has a problem with STRESS incontinence only. As you see, all of the accidents are related to movements or events that increase pressure on the bladder.

It is possible to experience leakage without the urge to void and without being able to identify a physical movement that caused the accident. If you found yourself wet and are unable to identify a reason, then you should not label that episode.

Go through all seven days of your first-week bladder diary and classify each accident. Mark each accident with a "U" or an "S." Try your best to label every accident.

Once you have finished labeling the accidents, review your entire diary and look at all of the accidents that you have labeled.

If all of your labeled accidents are marked with a "U," your problem may be URGE incontinence.

If all of your labeled accidents are marked with an "S," your problem may be STRESS incontinence.

If you have labeled some accidents with a "U" and some with an "S," your problem may be MIXED incontinence.

Circle your working diagnosis here, based on your first-week bladder diary:

URGE   STRESS   MIXED

Now, let's establish your final working diagnosis by comparing your diagnosis based on your answers to the Quick Quizzes and your diagnosis based on your first-week bladder diary. If your two working diagnoses are the same, then this is your final working diagnosis. If your two working diagnoses are different, then your final working diagnosis is MIXED incontinence.

Circle your final working diagnosis here:

URGE   STRESS   MIXED

At the lower right corner of each page in your first-week bladder diary, you will find a line for the total number of accidents. On that line place the total number of accidents (small or large, labeled or unlabeled) for that day. Do the same for each day.

Now fill in the number for each day and add them up:

Day #1   _____

Day #2   _____

Day #3   _____

Day #4   _____

Day #5   _____

Day #6   _____

Day #7   _____

_____

Total number of
accidents for
the first week   _____

Now that you have your final working diagnosis and you know the total number of accidents per week, you are ready to share this information with your doctor.

Call Your Doctor

Call your doctor now and make an appointment. Making an appointment to discuss your problem with your doctor is a big step. Some people do not seek help because they feel that their doctor won't understand what they are going through and won't be able to help them. There are also people who stay away from doctors because they fear what will happen if they reveal their problem with bladder control. A woman whose neighbor had surgery for incontinence might fear that she will be told to have surgery also. An elderly man who lives alone might fear that he will be placed in a nursing home. Fear should not prevent you from seeing a doctor. Surgery is an elective procedure. That is, you decide whether you want it. Furthermore, incontinence is never the only reason that an elderly person enters a nursing home. A medical evaluation will give you information about your condition that will allow you to make an informed decision regarding treatment.

What Kind of Doctor Should I Visit?

Go to your family doctor first. Your family physician knows you and your physical condition. For this reason, your family doctor is best able to conduct an initial evaluation and determine whether you need to be evaluated by a specialist.

If your family doctor does not have experience treating urinary incontinence, ask if there is a continence clinic or a continence specialist in your area. Health professionals who are most likely to be knowledgeable about incontinence are

- geriatricians: physicians who specialize in treating older adults

- gynecologists: physicians who specialize in the reproductive and urinary systems of women

- urologists: physicians who specialize in the urinary systems of men and women and the reproductive system of men

- nurse practitioners and nurses who specialize in incontinence, urology, gynecology, or the treatment of older adults.

Other professionals who may also be knowledgeable about incontinence include psychologists, physical therapists, occupational therapists, enterostomal therapists, social workers, and doctors who specialize in rehabilitation medicine. If you go to a continence clinic, you may be evaluated by a team consisting of several professionals who specialize in incontinence.

If you don't have a family doctor, talk to your friends or call your county or state medical society, your local hospital, or the closest university medical center. Ask if there is a continence clinic or a continence specialist in your area.

Throughout the rest of this book, we will use the term "doctor" to represent all health care professionals, although clearly there are a number of highly trained, nonphysician health care professionals who specialize in the evaluation and treatment of urinary incontinence.

Write the day, date, and time of your doctor's appointment here:

day	date	time

Read the rest of this chapter before you see your doctor. It will give you a better understanding of urinary incontinence and of your type of incontinence in particular. This will help you when you discuss your problem with your doctor.

The Urinary System

The urinary system is made up of four parts: the kidneys, the ureters, the bladder, and the urethra (see figs. 6 and 7). Together these organs produce, store, and eliminate urine—a normal waste product of the body.

The function of the kidneys is to filter blood continually. They separate elements that the body needs from waste products. These waste products combine with excess water to form urine. The kidneys are connected to the bladder by means of two narrow tubes called ureters. Urine flows down the ureters into the bladder. The bladder is a muscular organ that has two functions: to store urine and to empty urine. The urethra is a narrow tube that connects the bladder to the outside of the body. The opening of the urethra is at the end of the penis in men and just in front of the vagina in women.

The muscles and tissue of the pelvic floor help control the act of urinating. The pelvic floor is a sling of muscles and other tissues that supports the pelvic organs and their contents, including the bladder and urethra, the bowel, and, in women, the vagina and uterus (see figs. 8 and 9). The tissues of the pelvic floor are attached to bones on the front, the rear, and the sides of the lower pelvis.

In men, there are two openings in the pelvic floor: the urethra and the anus (the opening to the rectum) (see fig. 10). In women, there are three openings: the urethra, the vagina, and the anus (see fig. 11). Muscles of the pelvic floor that surround the urethra and the anus form sphincters. The urethral sphincter assists in the control of urine. It can be voluntarily relaxed to allow urine to flow out through the urethra, or it can be contracted to prevent the flow of urine.

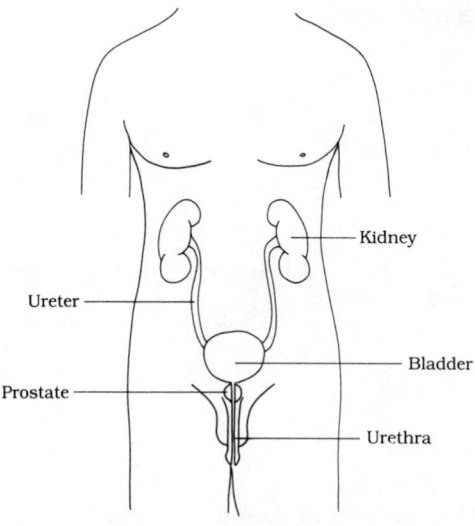

Figure 6. Front View of the Male Urinary System

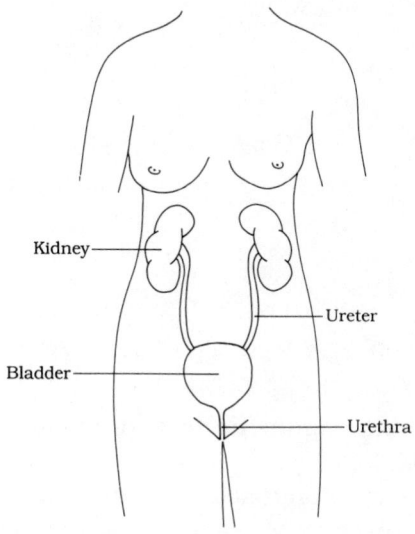

Figure 7. Front View of the Female Urinary System

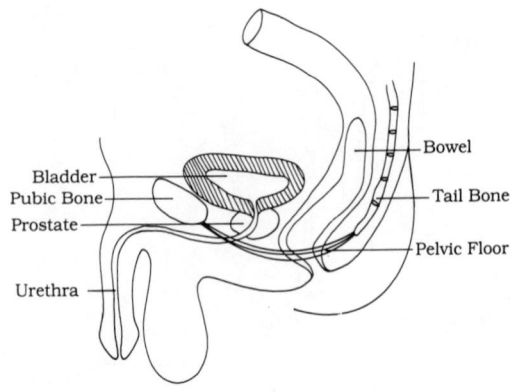

Figure 8. Side View of the Male Pelvis

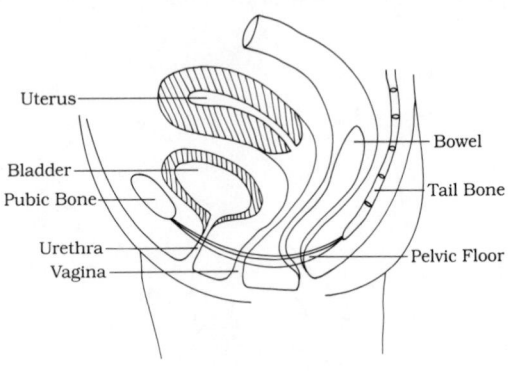

Figure 9. Side View of the Female Pelvis

Similarly, the anal sphincter helps to control the passage of stool and gas.

The prostate is a donut-shaped gland that surrounds the urethra between the bladder and the pelvic floor (see figs. 6 and 8). It is present only in men, and its primary function is to contribute fluid to semen.

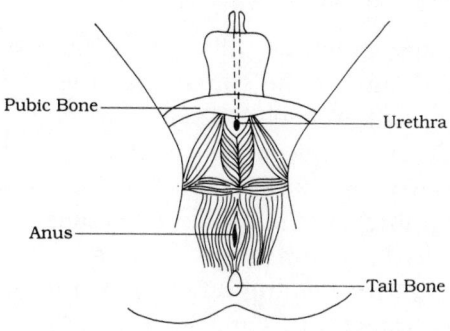

Figure 10. Male Pelvic Floor from Below (with Penis and Scrotum Raised), Showing Pelvic Floor Muscles

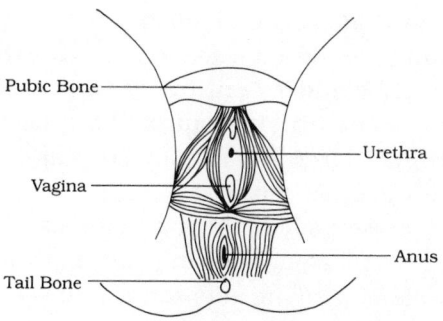

Figure 11. Female Pelvic Floor from Below, Showing Pelvic Floor Muscles

How the Bladder Works

As the bladder gradually fills with urine, the bladder expands and signals the spinal cord that it is getting increasingly full. When the signal reaches a certain intensity, the person becomes aware that the bladder is filling. This causes a feeling of fullness or pressure.

Bladder filling continues until it reaches a critical point, when the spinal cord signals the bladder to empty. This is the voiding reflex. This reflex activates the bladder muscle to contract and force urine out through the urethra. Thus, because of the voiding reflex, the bladder can empty without any connection to the brain, as it does in babies.

To *control* when the bladder empties, there must be a connection to the brain and the person must *learn* to control the voiding reflex. Ordinarily, this learning takes place during early childhood. During the process of toilet training, children learn to keep this reflex from emptying their bladders until they can reach a bathroom. They also learn to control the muscles of the pelvic floor. These muscles help by keeping the urethra closed until it is time to void.

Once a toilet is reached, the muscles surrounding the urethra can be relaxed, allowing the urethra to open. Then the bladder contracts and forces urine out through the urethra. Controlling when and where you void is a learned process. *Continence is a learned behavior.*

Categories of Incontinence

Bladder control is a complex series of events. If the process is to proceed correctly, the brain, the spinal cord, the urinary system, and the pelvic floor must all be in working order. Any disease or defect that affects any of these systems can produce incontinence.

There are two major categories of incontinence: acute incontinence and persistent incontinence.

Acute incontinence comes on suddenly and is usually caused by a new illness or condition. Some common causes of acute incontinence are

- irritation or inflammation
  - —of the bladder (cystitis)
  - —of the urethra (urethritis)
  - —of the vagina (vaginitis)
  - —of the prostate (prostatitis)

- medications
  - —diuretics (water pills) that increase the production of urine and fill the bladder more rapidly
  - —sleeping pills and sedatives that relax muscles and decrease awareness of the need to void
  - —decongestants that tighten the pelvic floor muscles and make it more difficult to void
  - —antidepressant drugs that relax the bladder and prevent it from contracting properly

- fecal impaction (large mass of stool in the rectum) that blocks or irritates the bladder

- confusion related to illness

- depression

- inability to move about due to illness

Acute incontinence is often easily reversed with appropriate treatment of the condition that caused it. Your doctor will help you determine whether you have acute incontinence by looking for reversible causes and then recommending treatment.

Persistent incontinence develops gradually over time or remains after other illnesses or conditions have been treated.

Types and Causes of Persistent Incontinence

There are six major types of persistent incontinence:

- urge incontinence
- stress incontinence
- mixed incontinence
- overflow incontinence
- total incontinence
- functional incontinence

Urge, stress, and mixed incontinence are the most common, together accounting for more than 80 percent of all incontinence.

Urge Incontinence: A Problem of the Bladder

Urge incontinence is also known as bladder instability, unstable bladder, uninhibited bladder, spastic bladder, irritable bladder, detrusor instability, motor instability, detrusor hyperreflexia, or neurogenic bladder. The problem is that the bladder misbehaves. It contracts and forces urine out of the body at the wrong times or in the wrong places because the voiding reflex is not being controlled properly. People with urge incontinence are unable to prevent the bladder from emptying before they can reach a bathroom. They are voiding too soon. Typically, urge incontinence is characterized by large accidents.

This inability to prevent urination can be caused by problems of the nervous system such as stroke, dementia, Parkinson's disease, multiple sclerosis, or spinal cord injury. It can also be caused by irritation or inflammation of the bladder or urethra due to conditions such as infection, thinning of the tissues of the urethra, fecal (stool) impaction, or enlargement of the prostate gland. Very often, a cause for urge incontinence cannot be found.

Stress Incontinence: A Problem of the Pelvic Floor

Stress incontinence is also known as sphincter insufficiency, sphincter incompetence, urethral insufficiency, or urethral incompetence. It is the loss of urine that occurs with a sudden rise in pressure in the abdomen (belly) from coughing, sneezing, lifting, or other physical activity. The increased pressure in the abdomen presses on the bladder. Urine escapes from the bladder not because of any defect in the bladder itself but because the urethra or pelvic floor is not working right. The urethra does not stay closed tightly enough to hold back urine during physical exertion. This happens because of weakness or damage to the muscles and other tissues that support the bladder and surround the urethra.

In women with stress incontinence, the tissues of the pelvic floor lose their ability to support the bladder and other pelvic organs properly. As a result, the pelvic organs may sag or drop into a lower position. When the bladder drops, it can produce a cystocele, which is a bulging of the bladder into the space occupied by the vagina. Similarly, a rectocele is the bulging of the rectum into the vagina. When support for the uterus is lost, it sags down into the vagina and is known as a uterine prolapse. All of these conditions are indicators of pelvic floor relaxation and can be diagnosed by pelvic examination.

Sometimes incontinence is blamed on a cystocele or rectocele. In fact, stress incontinence is not caused by the cystocele or rectocele but by weakness in the pelvic floor tissues. Cystoceles and rectoceles can be readily repaired surgically. However, the repair of a cystocele or rectocele may not improve incontinence. Surgery sometimes creates incontinence in a person who previously had normal bladder control.

In women, one major cause of stress incontinence is damage to the supporting tissues of the pelvic floor caused by pregnancy and childbirth. During pregnancy, the constant weight of the growing fetus exerts pressure on the pelvic floor, causing the tissues to stretch and sag. Likewise, during childbirth, the tissues are stretched and sometimes torn as the infant passes through the vagina.

As women age and pass through menopause (the "change of life"), their ovaries gradually produce less estrogen, a hormone that regulates the reproductive system. If a woman has a hysterectomy in which her ovaries are removed as well as the uterus, then her estrogen level drops rapidly. Without sufficient estrogen, the tissues of the vaginal area (including the pelvic floor muscles and urethra) may become thin and weak.

Stress incontinence is uncommon in men. When it does occur, the most frequent cause is injury to the urethra from a surgical procedure, such as a prostatectomy.

Can obesity cause stress incontinence? The evidence is inconclusive. However, it seems sensible to think that extra weight bears down on the pelvic floor and does result in stretching and sagging of tissues. Many people report that their bladder problem got worse when they gained weight or improved as they lost those extra pounds.

Mixed Incontinence: A Dual Problem

Many people have accidents in which they have a strong urge to void but cannot reach the toilet in time, *as well as* accidents with activities that cause increased abdominal pressure, such as coughing, sneezing, or lifting heavy objects. These people have mixed incontinence, with elements of both urge and stress incontinence.

Overflow Incontinence:
A Problem of Bladder Emptying

In overflow incontinence, the bladder cannot empty completely. It fills up and remains full, and excess urine that cannot fit in the bladder flows over and dribbles out through the urethra. Overflow incontinence occurs either because the bladder fails to contract properly or because the urethra is partially blocked.

Inability of the bladder to contract (called an atonic or acontractile bladder) means that there is a problem with the nerves that control the bladder. Usually, the cause is an injury to the spinal cord, diabetes that damages nerves, or some other problem of the nervous system. Such bladders hold very large volumes of urine, yet the person feels no desire to void.

The urethra can be blocked or obstructed in several ways. In men, the most common source of obstruction is an enlarged prostate.

Beginning in middle age, it is normal for the prostate to enlarge. This enlargement can be due to prostate cancer, but more commonly the cause is benign (noncancerous) growth, which is termed benign prostatic hypertrophy or hyperplasia (BPH). Some men have very little growth; in others, the prostate can grow to a size that causes problems with urination.

If the prostate enlarges too much, it can tighten around the urethra like a clamp around a garden hose. The effect is to pinch the urethra so that urine has a difficult time traveling through the narrowed passageway. When this happens, several problems can develop:

- difficulty getting the stream of urine started (hesitancy)

- a slow, weak, or interrupted stream of urine

- frequent voiding of small amounts of urine (frequency)

- pain or burning with voiding (dysuria)

- voiding at night (nocturia)

- an intense and often sudden need to void (urgency)

- dribbling after voiding

- the feeling or need to urinate again right after voiding (incomplete emptying)

- incontinence

If the prostate enlarges to the point where the urethra is completely blocked, this blockage can prevent urine from leaving the bladder (retention).

In men and women alike, any trauma to the urethra, as from a surgical procedure, can cause what is called a urethral stricture, where scar tissue narrows the urethra. Rarely, if a person has severe constipation, the flow of urine may be blocked. This problem is usually seen in institutionalized, severely disabled persons.

Another source of obstruction is called bladder-sphincter dyssynergia. Dyssynergia is a lack of coordination between the bladder and the pelvic floor muscles. Normally, when a person attempts to empty the bladder, the pelvic floor muscles relax, allowing the urethra to open. Then the bladder contracts and urine passes through. With dyssynergia, the pelvic floor muscles contract instead, clamping in on the urethra and interfering with the flow of urine. Thus, the bladder cannot empty completely. Dyssynergia is usually seen with problems of the nervous system, such as multiple sclerosis and spinal cord injuries.

Total Incontinence

Total incontinence is the complete loss of control and almost continual leakage of urine. It is rare. It may be caused by a bladder fistula, injury to the urethra, or an ectopic ureter.

A bladder fistula is a hole in the bladder. For example, when there is a hole in the walls that separate the bladder from the vagina, urine can leak continually from the bladder, through the vagina, and out of the body.

Total incontinence can also result from injury to the urethra during a surgical procedure or some other accident.

Occasionally, total incontinence is the result of a ureter that is not in the right place. Normally, the ureters enter the bladder well above the urethra. When the ureters enter too close to the urethra or if they empty directly into the urethra or the vagina, continual leakage of urine can result. This condition is called ectopic ureter.

Functional Incontinence

Functional incontinence is the loss of urine when a person is unable or unwilling to use the toilet appropriately. Using the bathroom is actually rather complicated, if you stop to think about it. Not only must you be able to reach the bathroom in time, you must also be able to get undressed and get on the toilet in time.

Functional incontinence, then, can be caused by any illness or problem that makes it hard to get around. For example, arthritis can be so painful and limiting that it keeps a person from reaching the toilet in time to avoid an accident. Muscle weakness, fatigue, problems with balance, broken bones, or joint problems can also make it difficult to get there, get undressed, and get on the toilet in time.

Disorders such as dementia that impair a person's memory can contribute to incontinence. Some people become confused and are not sure how to get to the bathroom or whether they need to use the bathroom. They may forget to go or forget what the toilet is used for.

Other people don't seem to mind that they are wet. This can happen when they receive more attention when they wet themselves than when they stay dry. Sometimes people become severely depressed and no longer care whether they are wet or dry. Depressed people may not even notice that they are wet.

Or the problem may be partly environmental, a result of living arrangements. For people who find it hard to get around anyway, uncomfortable toilet facilities might be enough to produce functional incontinence. Poor lighting, lack of privacy, and physical barriers can all increase the difficulty of reaching or using a toilet.

If you have functional incontinence because you have trouble getting around, you may find these suggestions helpful. Move your favorite chair or rearrange your bedroom so that your bed is closer to the bathroom. Make sure that the pathway to your bathroom is clear and well lit and that the bathroom door is left open. An elevated toilet seat or grab bars next to the toilet may make it easier to get on and off the toilet. A belt can be one more thing to fool with, one more obstacle between you and the toilet. Instead of a belt, wear clothing that is easy to remove, such as suspenders or slacks with an elastic waistband. Keep a urinal or bedpan handy, or put a portable commode chair in your bedroom or living room.

Now that you understand what urinary incontinence is and what might be causing your particular type of incontinence, it's time to prepare for your trip to the doctor. Read the next chapter—Step Three—*before* you go to your doctor, so that you'll know what to expect during your visit.

Your Trip to the Doctor

This book is *not* a substitute for your doctor. It is a guide to help you help yourself with your problem of bladder control. Visiting your doctor is an important step in helping yourself.

Why Is It Important to Visit Your Doctor?

Whether or not you consider your urine loss a problem and whether or not you want treatment, you should see your doctor for an evaluation. Urinary incontinence is a symptom of an underlying disorder, and sometimes that disorder can lead to more trouble if left untreated. Incontinence is a sign that "something isn't right." Don't ignore it.

The self-help strategies described later in this book may not be the most appropriate treatment for you. Sometimes the cause of incontinence is as simple as a bladder infection that can be treated with a few days of the proper medication. Certain types of incontinence— overflow or total incontinence—respond only to medical or surgical treatment. A visit to your doctor will reveal any easily reversible cause of incontinence, as well as any type that requires immediate medical or surgical treatment.

Preparing for Your Visit

Your doctor will have many questions to ask you about your problem. You may want to prepare for this by gathering important facts before you go to your appointment. You may find figure 12 helpful in organizing the necessary background information.

1. Appointment. Write in the day, date, and time of your appointment. This information should already be recorded on page 37 in Step Two.

2. Your Final Working Diagnosis. Write the final working diagnosis that you reached in Step Two on page 35.

3. Allergies. List any medications to which you have had any kind of reaction.

4. Medications. Make a list of all medications that you are taking, both prescription and over-the-counter drugs, including aspirin and cold preparations. Write the name, strength, and how often you take each medicine. If you are in doubt whether something counts as a medication, put it on the list.

5. Current Medical Problems. List all medical problems for which you are taking medications or are seeing a doctor.

6. Operations. List every operation you have had in your life.

7. Previous Urinary System History. Make a list of all events that may have affected your urinary system (such as childbirth), any illnesses you have had relating to this system (such as urinary tract infections or a history of blood in your urine), and any treatments or procedures you have had previously for your incontinence (such as surgery or

urethral dilatations). If you are a woman who is no longer having menstrual periods, write down how old you were when you stopped having periods.

8. Questions To Ask. Finally, write any questions that you may want to ask your doctor. We have provided several questions that everyone should ask.

What Will Your Doctor Do?

Different doctors will use different styles and methods to evaluate incontinence. Depending on individual training and unique experience, your doctor will make decisions about the best way to explore your problem. Your entire evaluation may not be completed in just one visit. Also, if your doctor intends to refer you to a continence specialist, your doctor may not perform the entire evaluation.

This section will introduce you to most of the commonly used procedures that you might encounter when you visit your doctor. Remember, each doctor approaches this problem a little differently.

The purpose of your evaluation is to identify the type and cause of your incontinence. Your initial evaluation should include an interview, a physical examination, a test of your urine, and a measurement of how well you are emptying your bladder. Your doctor may also do some blood tests.

The Interview

During your visit, your doctor will start by talking to you about your problem and may ask general questions about your health and past illnesses. The information

1. Appointment (day/date/time):

_____

2. Your final working diagnosis:

_____

3. Allergies to medication:
Name and reaction you had

_____

_____

_____

_____

_____

_____

4. Medications:

Name of medication	Strength	How often you take it
_____	_____	_____
_____	_____	_____
_____	_____	_____
_____	_____	_____
_____	_____	_____

5. Current medical problems:

_____

_____

_____

_____

_____

_____

Figure 12. Information for Your Doctor

6. Operations:

_____

_____

_____

_____

_____

_____

_____

7. Previous urinary system history:

_____

_____

_____

_____

_____

8. Questions to ask:

a. What type of urinary incontinence do I have?

b. What is the cause of my urinary incontinence?

c. What treatments are available for my type of urinary incontinence? What are the risks of these treatments? What are the side-effects of these treatments?

_____

_____

_____

_____

_____

_____

that you have gathered on figure 12 will provide most of the necessary answers.

Be prepared for the following questions specifically regarding your incontinence. You will find it helpful to review your first-week bladder diary with your doctor. The diary will answer many of these questions:

- When did your problem start?

- How did it start (did it come on suddenly or develop gradually over the years)?

- Has your condition improved or worsened over time?

- How often do you lose urine?

- How much urine do you lose during an accident?

- What causes you to lose urine?

- How often do you urinate during the day?

- How often do you urinate during the night (nocturia)?

- What is your fluid-intake pattern (what, how much, and when do you drink during the day)?

- Do you wear any padding or other form of protection?

- How does your bladder problem affect your activities?

- How does it affect the way you feel?

- Where are the bathrooms located in your house or workplace?

- What are your bowel habits? Do you suffer from constipation or soiling?

- When you urinate, do you have any of these problems:
    —an intense and often sudden need to void (urgency)
    —difficulty getting the stream of urine started (hesitancy)
    —a slow, weak, or interrupted stream of urine
    —frequent voiding of small amounts of urine (frequency)
    —pain or burning with voiding (dysuria)
    —dribbling after voiding
    —the feeling or need to urinate again right after voiding (incomplete emptying)
    —blood in your urine (hematuria)

Your doctor may also test your memory, as well as ask you questions about how you are feeling in general (your sleeping, eating, and sexual habits and if you get enjoyment out of your life).

Many people do not like to talk about bladder problems or emotional difficulties. If you are one of these people, you'll find that it helps to say that you are embarrassed. Doctors understand these feelings and will help you to speak frankly and accurately. It is important that you do because, based on your answers, your doctor will decide whether you have acute or persistent incontinence. Your answers will also provide clues to the type of incontinence that you have and what may be causing it. Therefore, you should answer all questions accurately.

If you feel that your doctor has the wrong impression of your problem, say so. Then help your doctor to understand exactly what happens to you. For example, it is very important for your doctor to understand how much urine you lose when you have an accident. "A little bit" might mean one or two drops to one person, but soaking only one pad to another. It is very easy to get the wrong impression when a person is not specific, so be as descriptive as possible. This will allow your doctor to understand your problem clearly.

The Physical Examination

After taking a medical history, your doctor will perform abdominal, pelvic, rectal, and neurological examinations. Your bladder should be full when the examination is started, so try not to void after you leave your house to go to the doctor.

When your doctor examines your abdomen (belly), it will be to look for an enlarged bladder or a mass, which may suggest that overflow incontinence is the problem. If the area over your bladder is tender when your doctor presses on it, this soreness may indicate that your bladder is enlarged.

With women, your doctor will then perform a pelvic examination. A speculum will be inserted into your vagina to look for any discharge or irritation that might suggest infection (vaginitis). Don't douche before your appointment, as this may temporarily wash away these important clues. Your doctor will also look for evidence of thinning of the vaginal walls, which may contribute to incontinence, as well as for a cystocele, rectocele, or uterine prolapse—all of which suggest weakness of the pelvic floor. The doctor will also look for a fistula or an ectopic ureter emptying into your vagina. Examining by hand, the doctor will again feel for any masses and may ask you to squeeze your vagina around the examining finger.

In both men and women, a rectal examination will be done to judge the muscle tone of your anal sphincter and its strength by asking you to squeeze around the examining finger. The doctor will feel for any masses or fecal impaction. You will also be tested for normal feeling around your anus. In men, the doctor will pay special attention to the size and firmness of the prostate gland, as well as to any tenderness you may feel during the examination.

While you are still on the examining table, your doctor may ask you to cough, looking to see if you lose urine. If you do not leak while coughing, you may be asked to stand up and cough again, bounce on your heels, walk, or bend over. Don't be embarrassed if you leak urine during this part of the examination. What makes you leak is exactly what you want to find out, after all. These actions are called "stress maneuvers" or a "stress test" because they may cause you to leak urine if you have stress incontinence.

Next, your doctor may perform a neurological examination, testing the strength in your legs and your reflexes. Your doctor may also check to see whether you are able to tell when your legs are being touched with a pin. During this part of the examination, your doctor is looking for evidence of any problems with the nervous system that may be causing your incontinence, such as Parkinson's disease or diseases of the spinal cord.

The Urine Test

You may be asked to provide a "midstream" or "clean-catch" urine specimen. To do this, you will be given several moist pads and a sterile cup. If you are a woman, expose the opening of your urethra by separating your labia (lips) with your thumb and index finger. If you are an uncircumcised man, pull back your foreskin. Keep your labia separated or your foreskin pulled back throughout the collection. Next, clean the area around the urethral opening with the moist pads, wiping in a front-to-back or top-to-bottom motion. Then start to urinate in the toilet. Without stopping the stream, catch some of your urine in the cup. Remove the cup before you finish, and finish urinating in the toilet. When urine is collected in this careful way, your doctor can be sure that the urine sample is not contaminated with bacteria from outside your body.

You may be asked simply to urinate into a cup. You can do this without special instructions.

Your urine will be examined under a microscope to check for any abnormalities. Your doctor will be looking for white blood cells, red blood cells, and bacteria. If white blood cells, bacteria, or both are seen, this may mean that you have a urinary tract infection and will need treatment with an antibiotic. In that case, your doctor may send part of your urine sample for a urine culture test to see which particular bacteria are present.

If your doctor sees only red blood cells, you may be asked to provide another urine specimen later that day or on another day. Blood in the urine is known as hematuria. Hematuria sometimes occurs for unknown reasons, and it may have no consequences. However, hematuria may also be a sign of serious illness and should be investigated with further tests. If you are a woman who is menstruating on the day of your appointment, be sure to tell your doctor. The doctor may want to postpone your urine test until after your period is over because blood from your vagina can get into your urine sample.

When you return to the examination room, your doctor may again examine your abdomen briefly. Your postvoid residual urine will then be checked.

The Postvoid Residual Urine

To determine whether you are emptying your bladder completely, your doctor will perform a simple procedure called bladder catheterization. While you are lying on your back, your genital area will be cleaned. Your doctor will pass a sterile, narrow tube (catheter) through your urethra into your bladder. When the catheter enters your bladder, it allows the drainage of any urine that was left in your bladder after you finished urinating. It is normal for a small amount of urine to remain in the bladder after voiding, but large amounts indicate that the bladder is not emptying properly. Perhaps your bladder is not contracting strongly enough, or perhaps there is a blockage of the urethra—both suggesting overflow as the type of incontinence. If your doctor has difficulty inserting the catheter, that also suggests blockage of the urethra, usually from enlargement of the prostate in men or a urethral stricture.

Bladder catheterization takes only a few minutes. You may feel some discomfort when the catheter is put in or removed. Also, there is a very small risk (1 to 2 percent) that the procedure may cause an infection in your bladder.

Blood Tests

Your doctor may want to take a sample of your blood to test for sugar, calcium, and how well your kidneys are working [creatinine or blood urea nitrogen (BUN)]. An elevated blood sugar or calcium level can cause increased production of urine and lead to incontinence. If your kidneys are not working properly, this could also lead to an increased production of urine.

After your initial evaluation, your doctor may be able

to describe the type and cause of your incontinence and recommend appropriate treatment. However, if your doctor needs more information to make a diagnosis, further evaluation and testing will be recommended. A number of tests can be performed to provide this extra information. Some of these tests can be done right in your doctor's office. Other tests require special experience and equipment, so your doctor may need to refer you to another health care professional.

Be sure to ask your doctor to explain these additional tests. Why are they desirable? What will the results tell the doctor? Find out who will perform the tests, where they will be done, how they are done, and what risks are involved.

In Appendix A, you will find an alphabetical listing of other tests that may be suggested to you. Some of these may be called urodynamic tests because they test how the bladder and urethra work. Many of these tests are used commonly in the evaluation of incontinence; others are used less frequently. Appendix A is a guide to these tests. It includes a description of each test, what information it provides, and any risks and special instructions.

After you have seen your doctor and after all test results have been received, you and your doctor will discuss the diagnosis. Now is the time to ask the questions that you have written on figure 12. After your doctor has described the type and cause of your incontinence, it is time to discuss your treatment.

Based on past experience with various treatments, your doctor will recommend a treatment for you. This recommendation will be based on your general health, your specific health problems, your type of incontinence, the cause of your incontinence, the medications you are taking, and your life situation.

For any given type of incontinence, there is more than one method of treatment. The major treatment methods are

- behavioral training procedures
- medications
- surgery
- bladder catheterization

In Appendix B, you will find a list of treatment options that may be offered to you. These options are all accepted methods for treating urinary incontinence. Appendix B is a guide to these treatment options. It includes an explanation of each treatment along with its specific usages and risks. All of the methods described have been helpful for many people with incontinence.

You would be wise to learn about all of your treatment options and to ask your doctor about them *before* you make a decision. Discuss all of the treatments that might be appropriate for you. Ask about the advantages and disadvantages of each treatment. Ask specifically about any risks that might be involved. Finally, when your doctor recommends a treatment, be sure to ask for an explanation of the reasons for that choice and why the doctor prefers it over other treatments. If you are uncomfortable with your doctor's recommendation, you may wish to get a second opinion.

Remember, the final decision is yours. In making this decision, it is important that you understand

- no single method is right for everyone
- no single method works for everyone
- every method has advantages

- every method has disadvantages

- nobody can predict how you will respond to any given treatment

If you asked five different doctors, it is possible that you would receive five different opinions. This is not because the doctors don't know what they are doing. It's because knowledge about incontinence is not so far advanced that there is agreement on which treatment is best for whom. Choosing the best treatment for you is not an exact science. Therefore, we recommend that you be prepared to try a second treatment if the first does not work.

When you go to the doctor, remember to take this book with you. Your first-week bladder diary at the end of Step One, your answers to the Quick Quizzes and your final working diagnosis in Step Two, and the information that you have gathered on figure 12 earlier in Step Three will all be very helpful to your doctor.

Now you know what to expect from your visit to the doctor, what additional tests may be suggested, and what treatments are available to you.

When all of your questions have been answered and you have all of the information you need, make your choice.

Taking Control

You've completed and interpreted your first-week bladder diary, so you know more about your problem with urinary incontinence. You've seen your doctor, you've had an evaluation, you've discussed all of the treatments available to you, and you've decided to try this behavioral treatment program, which combines pelvic floor muscle exercises and new strategies to prevent urine loss. Now it is time for you to take control of your bladder instead of allowing your bladder to control you.

This behavioral treatment program consists of carefully developed methods based on the extensive clinical experiences of physicians, nurses, physical therapists, psychologists, and other professionals. These methods have been applied with success by thousands of men and women with urge incontinence, stress incontinence, and mixed incontinence. These methods are safe and without the side-effects and risks that other treatments may have. And these methods require no special equipment or procedures. You already have all the special materials you will need—this book.

Pelvic Floor Muscles

The pelvic floor muscles are a group of muscles that support the bladder and urethra, the bowel, and, in women, the vagina and the uterus. These muscles surround the urethra, the vagina, and the anus. It is these pelvic floor muscles that you learn to squeeze to keep the urethra closed and to relax to allow the urethra to open. Usually, the pelvic floor muscles act as a group, squeezing and relaxing together.

The pelvic floor muscle exercises that you will learn are similar to Kegel exercises, named after Dr. A. H. Kegel, the gynecologist who developed them. As early as 1948, Dr. Kegel found that these exercises were effective in the treatment of women with stress incontinence. Many men and women have heard of these exercises and have tried them. Unfortunately, many have not found them helpful, for at least three reasons. First, some people never locate the right muscles to exercise. Second, they then exercise the wrong muscles and may even increase their incontinence as a result. Third, they give up too soon. Even when the right muscles are identified, people tend to give up after only a few days, well before the exercises can take effect.

We will begin by helping you find your pelvic floor muscles. Then we will outline a program of exercises to strengthen your pelvic floor muscles. Most important, we will help you learn how to use them the right way.

Locating Your Pelvic Floor Muscles

There are several ways to find your pelvic floor muscles. Each one is described separately. You should be alone in a quiet place where you can concentrate and experiment. After you read each technique, take several minutes to try it. If the first technique doesn't work for you, go on to the next. It doesn't matter which technique you use to find your pelvic floor muscles because the muscles tend to work as a group. So squeezing any one of the pelvic floor muscles indicates that the others are working too. Every person is unique, and different techniques work for different people.

Technique #1

Go to the toilet and start to void. Once the stream of urine has started, try to stop it. Close your eyes and think about trying to stop the stream of urine. If you can slow the stream of urine, even slightly, you are using the right muscles.

Technique #2

If you are a woman, lie down and insert a finger into your vagina. Try to squeeze around your finger with your vaginal muscles. You should be able to feel the sensation in your vagina, and you may also be able to feel the pressure on your finger. If you can, you are using the right muscles. If you cannot detect any movement with one finger, try two fingers.

Technique #3

If you are a man, stand in front of a mirror and watch your penis. Try to make your penis move up and down without moving the rest of your body. If you can, you are using the right muscles.

Technique #4

Everyone, at one time or another, has been in a crowded room and felt as if he or she were going to pass gas. Imagine that this is happening to you. Try to squeeze the muscles at your anus that would prevent you from passing gas. If you feel a "pulling" sensation at the anus, you are using the right muscles.

Technique #5

Insert the tip of a finger into your anus and try to squeeze your finger as if you are holding back a bowel movement. You should be able to feel the sensation in your anus as well as the pressure on your finger. If you can, you are using the right muscles.

You may not find your pelvic floor muscles immediately. Many people have to take their time with this. Remember, you are searching for muscles that you may not have been aware of before. Your muscles may be weak, so for now your goal is only to locate your pelvic floor muscles.

Don't Use the Wrong Muscles!

When trying to find a new muscle, especially a weak one, most people tighten other muscles too. Some people clench their fists or teeth, hold their breath, or make a face. None of these helps. It is very tempting to use other muscles, especially stronger ones, to support smaller, weaker muscles such as the pelvic floor muscles. However, using other muscles interferes with learning how to use the right ones. It is best just to relax your body as much as possible and concentrate on your pelvic floor muscles.

The most commonly used "wrong muscles" are the muscles of the abdomen (belly). Most people who are learning to control their pelvic floor muscles tense their belly muscles at the same time. This happens so often that the muscles may seem to be connected. They are not. It is very important to separate the muscle groups and to keep your abdominal muscles relaxed while you squeeze your pelvic floor muscles. When tightened, abdominal muscles raise the pressure in your bladder and actually make it more likely that you will leak urine. Abdominal muscles tend to push urine out of the bladder instead of holding it in.

To avoid using your abdominal muscles, rest your hand lightly on your abdomen as you are squeezing your pelvic floor muscles. Do you feel your belly tightening? If you do, relax and try again. Be sure that you do not feel any movement of your abdomen.

Are you holding your breath? If you are, you are probably using your abdominal muscles. First, relax completely and notice how you are breathing for a few moments. Then, squeeze your pelvic floor muscles while you continue to breath normally. This will help to assure that you are not using your abdominal muscles because abdominal muscles are usually relaxed when you breathe.

The other set of "wrong muscles" are the muscles of the buttocks (bottom). To test whether you are also tightening your buttock muscles by mistake, squeeze your pelvic floor muscles while sitting in front of a mirror. If you see that your body is moving up and down slightly, you are also using your buttock muscles. When done properly, no one should be able to tell that you are squeezing your pelvic floor muscles—except you.

If you cannot find any of your pelvic floor muscles, consult your health care professional for assistance with this step. Once you have found the muscles, even if they are weak, read on.

Strengthening Your Pelvic Floor Muscles

Now that you have located your pelvic floor muscles and you are able to squeeze them without using your abdominal or buttock muscles, you are ready to begin your daily exercise program.

Daily exercise has two functions. First, exercise increases the *strength* of your pelvic floor muscles, so that they will be strong enough to prevent accidents. Second, through repeated practice you gain control over these muscles. Then you can use them *quickly* to prevent urine loss. These exercises are the mainstay of your program.

Learning pelvic floor muscle exercises may be difficult at first and may require more concentration than you expect. This is true for most new skills. Do you remember learning to drive a car? With a multitude of details to keep in mind, it is hard to imagine driving as automatically as most of us do. Well, learning to exercise pelvic floor muscles is also a skill. Rest assured that with persistence and continued practice, these exercises will become second nature. Soon you will find yourself doing them automatically.

If at any time you find yourself getting the wrong muscles involved, STOP! Rest for a moment and start again, using just your pelvic floor muscles. If you are tired and unable to stop using the wrong muscles, stop and rest! Go back to the exercises later in the day.

The Exercise

Each exercise consists of squeezing and then relaxing your pelvic floor muscles. Squeeze the muscles for three seconds and then relax the muscles for three seconds. The easiest way to do this is to squeeze and count slowly "1—2—3." Then relax and again count slowly "1—2—3." A squeeze and relax is considered one exercise. Do one exercise now.

Holding the muscles to a slow count of three is important for increasing muscle strength. Remember, squeeze and count slowly "1—2—3," then relax and again count slowly "1—2—3." Do another exercise. Make sure you hold the squeeze for the full three seconds.

As a shortcut, you may be tempted to squeeze the muscles but not take the time to relax in between squeezes. Wrong. You must allow the muscles to relax between squeezes so that they can rest before squeezing again. Take time to relax to the same count (1—2—3) as you squeeze (1—2—3). Now do two exercises. Make sure you relax completely between squeezes.

The exercises are best done in three positions: lying, sitting, and standing. Why in three positions? It is essential for you to feel comfortable using your pelvic floor muscles in all positions. The sensation that you will feel while squeezing is different when you are standing compared to when you are sitting or lying. More important, you may need to prevent leakage in any of these three positions, so you must have control over your pelvic floor muscles in all positions. Now practice one exercise in each position: lying, sitting, and standing.

Many people find that the standing position is the most difficult. Part of the problem is that you are less likely to feel the contraction of your muscles while you are standing. You may think that the muscles are not working properly when, in fact, they are working just fine. Keep trying. You will need your muscles in the standing position. Do one more exercise in the standing position.

The First Two Weeks

Do forty-five pelvic floor muscle exercises every day, divided into three sessions of fifteen exercises each. (Remember, each squeeze and relax counts as one exercise.) Do the exercises in each position every day: fifteen exercises lying, fifteen standing, and fifteen sitting. The exact time of day is not critical. What is critical is that you develop the habit of doing the exercises every day. You can make this happen by planning your exercise schedule in advance. Choose three times of day when you can be sure you will always have time to exercise.

In the beginning, you will need to set aside time to concentrate while you do the exercises. This time should be a quiet time, when you are alone with no disturbances. Each time should be associated with a cue that will remind you to practice. For example, you may want to exercise just before or just after each of your three meals. Any activity that you perform regularly on a daily basis can be used as a cue.

Plan now when you will set aside three times to do your exercises each day:

Lying session: _____

Standing session: _____

Sitting session: _____

Remember to do fifteen exercises at each session. Doing the exercises in sets of fifteen assures that the muscles are strengthened. Doing fewer exercises at each session, even if they total forty-five for the day, may not exercise the muscles adequately. If you tire before you reach fifteen, rest briefly and then finish the session.

Are you worried that it will take too much time? If

you are squeezing and relaxing to a slow count of three, a session of fifteen exercises will take you about one and a half minutes.

When you are counting "1—2—3" at the same time that you are counting exercises, you may lose track of how many exercises you have done. If this happens to you, you can set a timer for the total time you expect to be exercising. Since you will be squeezing and relaxing to a slow count of three, you should set the timer for one and a half minutes.

If you would like to do more than forty-five exercises each day, feel free to do so. Pelvic floor muscle exercises cannot hurt you—they can only help. In fact, most people who have overcome incontinence with this method report that they also exercise whenever they think about it throughout the day (in addition to their scheduled forty-five exercises). When it occurs to them, they simply squeeze their muscles a few times to keep in practice. Try to do three or four exercises whenever you stand up from a chair, when you stop at a red light, when you get into your car, when you find yourself standing in line at the bank or the grocery store, whenever the telephone rings. Squeezing your pelvic floor muscles whenever you think of them helps to make their use easier and more automatic in your daily life. No one will know that you are using them, except you.

Soon, after two weeks of exercise, you will find yourself able to hold the squeeze comfortably to a count of three for the full fifteen exercises.

Remember, your pelvic floor muscles are weak in the beginning. Like any other muscle, they need some time to gain strength. Many people give up after only several days of practice because they see no change. Pelvic floor muscles need more time. You will probably see improvement after the first two weeks, but the muscles may not reach their full potential for at least six months.

Start your first two weeks of exercise now. As you finish each session, check it off on the exercise calendars that follow. This will help you to keep track of your exercise schedule. Remember, you can always do more exercises whenever you think of it during the day.

First-Week Exercise Calendar

	Day 1	Day 2	Day 3	Day 4	Day 5	Day 6	Day 7
Lying	☐	☐	☐	☐	☐	☐	☐
Standing	☐	☐	☐	☐	☐	☐	☐
Sitting	☐	☐	☐	☐	☐	☐	☐

Second-Week Exercise Calendar

	Day 1	Day 2	Day 3	Day 4	Day 5	Day 6	Day 7
Lying	☐	☐	☐	☐	☐	☐	☐
Standing	☐	☐	☐	☐	☐	☐	☐
Sitting	☐	☐	☐	☐	☐	☐	☐

You are ready now—after only two weeks of exercise—to begin to use your pelvic floor muscles to prevent urinary accidents. Making the muscles strong is essential. Now you will learn how to use them.

The Third and Fourth Weeks

- If you have URGE incontinence, continue your pelvic floor muscle exercises every day and proceed now to the next section—"Controlling Urge Incontinence."

- If you have STRESS incontinence, continue your pelvic floor muscle exercises every day, skip the next section, and proceed now to page 82—"Controlling Stress Incontinence."

- If you have MIXED incontinence, you will need to read both sections. Continue your pelvic floor muscles exercises every day and read the next section—"Controlling Urge Incontinence"—now.

Controlling Urge Incontinence

Urge incontinence is the loss of urine when you have a strong urge or desire to void and are unable to make it to the bathroom in time.

Urge or urgency is a *feeling*—nothing more. It is an uncomfortable feeling that makes you want to empty your bladder. It may indicate that your bladder is full and ready to empty. On the other hand, your bladder may not be full but may be contracting and trying to empty anyway. The urge is a message from your bladder telling you to void. Do you have to obey?

You have probably heard the phrase, "When you gotta go, you gotta go." This implies that there is no choice. NOT TRUE. Immediate voiding is not necessary. The fact is that the urge feeling lets you know only that voiding is necessary, not that voiding must occur immediately. Your goal, of course, is not to void until you reach a toilet, something that may not be available right away. The normal bladder has learned to wait; your bladder has lost that ability. Improved control will be yours when you can retrain your bladder to wait.

Normal urge feelings come in waves (see fig. 13). First, you feel the urge a little. Then it grows, it peaks, and, finally, it subsides. People with urge incontinence have temporarily lost the ability to make urges subside, or they don't take the time to make urges subside. They are usually too busy rushing to the toilet when urgency is at its peak.

As the urgency feeling increases and voiding seems necessary, most people with urge incontinence rush to the toilet—believing that the faster they get there, the better. You may feel that it is only a matter of time before your bladder starts to empty but that you will be okay as long as you can "beat it" to the toilet. It may seem that rushing to the bathroom is the best thing— and the only thing—you can do.

Actually, *rushing* is the worst thing you can do. The rushing itself contributes to accidents for four reasons.

- Rushing jiggles your bladder, increasing your awareness of how full it feels and making the urgency worse.

- Movement can stimulate the bladder to contract and empty.

- Rushing puts extra abdominal pressure on the bladder and tends to push urine out.

- Rushing interferes with the concentration that you need to control your bladder.

Rushing *to the bathroom* is even worse. Getting to the bathroom just in time seems to be evidence that faster is better. Getting to the bathroom may seem like the best thing because you just barely make it there before you start to drip. Or you start dripping just before you reach the toilet. But think about it: It is no coincidence that you just make it to the bathroom as urgency reaches its peak. For a person with urge incontinence, it is the bathroom itself that makes the urge worse and contributes to the accident.

Approaching the toilet can be the most difficult time for anyone to control the bladder. Have you ever noticed that seeing a bathroom or even thinking about a bathroom makes you feel like you have to use it? That's exactly the problem. After many years of urinating in bathrooms, the bathroom has come to be associated with urination. You have been conditioned, so that the bathroom actually triggers your desire to urinate. Therefore, if you already have an urge to void, approaching the bathroom is likely to heighten the need to void and make incontinence a more likely event.

For a person with urge incontinence, the worst time to head for the bathroom is when you already have a strong urge to urinate (see fig. 14). The best time is *before* you get the urge or *after* you have successfully reduced or eliminated the urge to void.

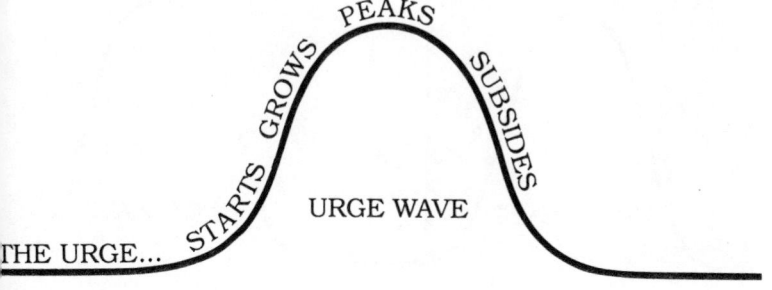

Figure 13. Urge Wave

You may think that the only way to relieve the uncomfortable feeling of urgency is to empty your bladder, but you will see that this is not so. Urges can come and go without your emptying the bladder; they are simply messages telling you that eventually you will need to void. Urges are not commands. They should function as an early warning system, getting you ready to find a place to void—*after* you have relaxed and suppressed the urge.

To reduce or eliminate the urge to void, you will use your pelvic floor muscles. When you start to feel the urge, squeeze your pelvic floor muscles quickly several times. Do not relax fully in between squeezes. Try this now.

Squeezing your pelvic floor muscles in this way sends a message to your bladder to stop contracting. As your bladder stops contracting and starts relaxing, the urge feeling subsides.

Then, once the urge to void has subsided, you have a safe period when the bladder is calm. This "calm period" is the best time to go to the bathroom.

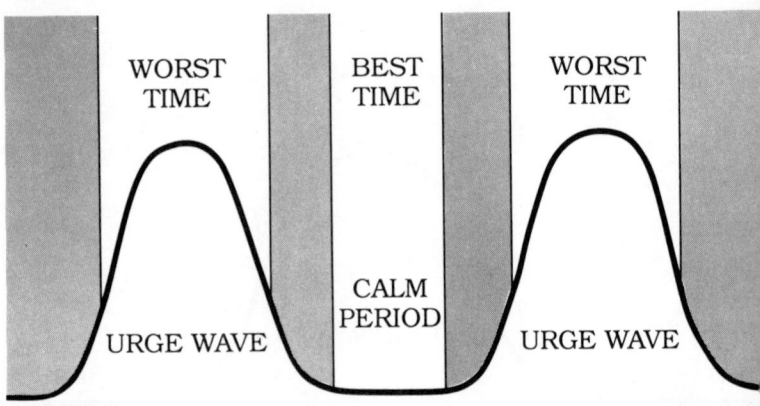

Figure 14. When to Void

Let's look at exactly what you should do when an urge feeling strikes. There are six simple steps to follow.

1. Stop what you are doing and stay put. Sit down when possible, or stand quietly. Remain very still. When you are still, it is easier to control your urge.

2. Squeeze your pelvic floor muscles quickly several times. Do not relax fully in between.

3. Relax the rest of your body. Take a few deep breaths to help you relax and let go of your tension.

4. Concentrate on suppressing the urge feeling.

5. Wait until the urge subsides.

6. Walk to the bathroom at a normal pace. Do not rush. Continue squeezing your pelvic floor muscles quickly while you walk.

For example, if you are out driving and you have a strong urge, follow these six simple steps. Then, stop at the next restroom, when the urge has subsided.

Be Prepared

Urgency often strikes when you least expect it. You can prepare for urgency by learning to anticipate when it will strike. Review your first-week bladder diary for all of the situations in which you had urge accidents. As you approach one of these situations, squeeze your pelvic floor muscles quickly several times. This may prevent your urge feeling from starting.

For example, many people note that the urge feeling strikes as they stand up from a sitting position. To prepare for this situation, squeeze your pelvic floor muscles quickly several times *before* you change positions. Then squeeze your pelvic floor muscles and hold that squeeze while you stand up. This approach allows you to maintain control through the process of rising to a standing position. In the morning when you awaken with a full bladder is also a good time to avoid accidents with this approach.

Start Safe

Before you have used these techniques, you may be skeptical and fearful of having an accident. Because these are new skills for you, it is possible that your first attempt won't work, perhaps not even your first few tries. It is important, therefore, to begin practicing these new approaches in a safe place, such as at home.

With continued practice, you will be able to suppress urgency, so that the urge feeling will diminish or go away. You may even be able to avoid the urge entirely. As you gain confidence, apply these techniques to other settings.

- If you have URGE incontinence, continue your pelvic floor muscle exercises every day and start to use these techniques. Proceed to page 85 and use the exercise calendars for the third and fourth weeks.

- If you have MIXED incontinence, continue your pelvic floor muscle exercises every day and start to use these techniques. Proceed now to the next section—"Controlling Stress Incontinence."

Controlling Stress Incontinence

Stress accidents are caused by physical activity or movements such as coughing, lifting, sneezing, jogging, or even standing up. These events cause increased pressure in your abdomen, which presses on your bladder. Urine escapes because your urethra, which is surrounded by the urethral sphincter (one of the pelvic floor muscles), is unable to stay closed tightly enough.

After two weeks of exercise, the strength of your pelvic floor muscles has improved. Now you will learn how to use them to prevent stress accidents.

The way to prevent stress incontinence is to squeeze your pelvic floor muscles just before and during whatever activities cause you to lose urine. Then relax. For example, as you are about to cough, squeeze your pelvic floor muscles. Keep squeezing them while you cough, then relax them when the coughing is over.

Certain activities, such as tennis or jogging, are extended activities. It is not possible to keep your pelvic floor muscles squeezed throughout the entire activity. In such cases, you can reduce leakage by squeezing during the most physically stressful moments, such as swinging the racket during tennis. During more sustained activities like jogging, you can reduce leakage by squeezing and relaxing your pelvic floor muscles off-and-on throughout the entire activity.

Your first-week bladder diary has made you aware of all of the events that cause you to have accidents. Review your diary now and make a list of all of the activities and movements that make you leak.

I leak urine when I:

_____	_____
_____	_____
_____	_____
_____	_____
_____	_____

Review this list several times. It will remind you of your "risky" times, the times when you will need to use your pelvic floor muscles to prevent accidents.

In addition to the times on your list, squeeze when you laugh, when you blow your nose, when you sneeze, and when you push or pull. Squeeze your pelvic floor muscles when you stand up from a chair or bed, when you climb stairs, and when you stoop to lift something. This will help you to develop the habit of squeezing your pelvic floor muscles whenever pressure inside your abdomen is high.

Helpful Hints

When you start using this technique, you may not remember to squeeze every time you engage in an activity or movement that causes you to leak. Don't worry; this is a common problem at first. It is normal when developing any new habit. If you forget to squeeze before and during an activity that causes you to leak, be sure to squeeze as soon as you remember. This will not prevent that accident, but it will help you develop the new habit. Once it is developed, it will become second nature to you. You will find yourself squeezing your muscles automatically.

Some things happen so suddenly or unexpectedly that there doesn't seem to be enough time to squeeze. You may be afraid that there will not be enough warning to be able to squeeze the muscles before you start to leak. You will find that, with a little practice, there is enough time. Most people know that there is enough time to cross their legs before they sneeze. If there is enough time to cross your legs, there is enough time to squeeze.

Let's Practice

Look at your list of events that cause you to lose urine. Pick one that you can perform at home, such as carrying a heavy object or coughing. Practice the technique for the first few times right now. Before you start the activity, squeeze your pelvic floor muscles. Keep squeezing as you perform the activity. After the activity is over, relax your pelvic floor muscles.

Don't give up if you fail the first few times you try to prevent accidents. Your progress will be gradual, and it will depend on how faithfully you exercise your muscles and how regularly you practice this technique. The more you exercise, the stronger and quicker your pelvic floor muscles will become. The more you practice squeezing during events that cause you to leak urine, the more familiar it will become. You will soon be squeezing those muscles without even thinking about it. Gradually, you will see fewer accidents and smaller accidents.

Continue your pelvic floor muscle exercises every day and start to use these techniques. Use the following exercise calendars for the third and fourth weeks.

Third-Week Exercise Calendar

	Day 1	Day 2	Day 3	Day 4	Day 5	Day 6	Day 7
Lying	☐	☐	☐	☐	☐	☐	☐
Standing	☐	☐	☐	☐	☐	☐	☐
Sitting	☐	☐	☐	☐	☐	☐	☐

Fourth-Week Exercise Calendar

	Day 1	Day 2	Day 3	Day 4	Day 5	Day 6	Day 7
Lying	☐	☐	☐	☐	☐	☐	☐
Standing	☐	☐	☐	☐	☐	☐	☐
Sitting	☐	☐	☐	☐	☐	☐	☐

You are ready now—after four weeks of exercise—to strengthen your pelvic floor muscles even more.

The Fifth through Tenth Weeks

In your daily exercise sessions over the next several weeks, you will need gradually to extend the time you squeeze and relax to a full ten seconds. The reason for this progression from three to ten seconds is to make sure that your pelvic floor muscles get stronger and can stay squeezed for a longer period. As the pelvic floor muscles become stronger, you will be able to do fifteen exercises consecutively, to a count of ten seconds each, without difficulty. This gradual progression will take place over the next three weeks. Remember that the ultimate goal is to squeeze for ten seconds and relax for ten seconds. Continue to use the techniques that you have learned to prevent accidents.

The Fifth Week

During the fifth week, you will increase the time you squeeze and relax to five seconds. Squeeze and count slowly "1—2—3—4—5," then relax and again count slowly "1—2—3—4—5." Each set of fifteen exercises should now take about two and a half minutes to complete. If you are using a timer to help you count exercises, set it for two and a half minutes.

Fifth-Week Exercise Calendar

	Day 1	Day 2	Day 3	Day 4	Day 5	Day 6	Day 7
Lying	☐	☐	☐	☐	☐	☐	☐
Standing	☐	☐	☐	☐	☐	☐	☐
Sitting	☐	☐	☐	☐	☐	☐	☐

The Sixth Week

During the sixth week, you will extend the time you squeeze and relax to eight seconds, a slow count of "1—2—3—4—5—6—7—8." Each set of fifteen exercises will now take about four minutes to complete.

Sixth-Week Exercise Calendar

	Day 1	Day 2	Day 3	Day 4	Day 5	Day 6	Day 7
Lying	☐	☐	☐	☐	☐	☐	☐
Standing	☐	☐	☐	☐	☐	☐	☐
Sitting	☐	☐	☐	☐	☐	☐	☐

The Seventh Week

Now you are ready to increase the time you squeeze and relax to a full ten seconds. Each set of fifteen exercises should now take about five minutes.

Seventh-Week Exercise Calendar

	Day 1	Day 2	Day 3	Day 4	Day 5	Day 6	Day 7
Lying	☐	☐	☐	☐	☐	☐	☐
Standing	☐	☐	☐	☐	☐	☐	☐
Sitting	☐	☐	☐	☐	☐	☐	☐

After seven weeks of exercise, your pelvic floor muscles are even stronger. Now when you squeeze your pelvic floor muscles, you will be better able to prevent accidents.

For women, there is often a bonus. The pelvic floor muscles are those that contract during orgasm. Many women find that these exercises have made them more sexually responsive, even as early as the seventh week. Your partner will also be delighted by your new ability to squeeze your pelvic floor muscles around his penis during intercourse. For men, strengthening the pelvic floor muscles can help achieve firmer erections, greater ejaculatory control, and more powerful orgasms.

The Eighth Week

After seven weeks of practice, the exercises will require less effort, and you will no longer need to set aside special times to concentrate on them. Instead, you can do the exercises while you do other activities in your daily life. For example, you may want to do your standing exercises in the shower. Your sitting exercises may be done while sitting in a chair reading or watching television. You may want to do the exercises lying down before you get out of bed in the morning or before you fall asleep at night.

Doing the exercises at the same time and along with something else that you do every day will help you to remember to do them regularly. You want to build these exercises into your life, so you never have to think about them. You will simply do them, in the automatic way you brush your teeth. This is where many people fail. A new habit is sometimes hard to start but, once in the swing, it becomes second nature.

Remember, the activities that you choose should be things you do every day, all year round. Here are some ideas to help you get started. Do fifteen exercises

- when you shower
- while you walk the dog
- when you brush your teeth
- as you watch television
- while you read in bed
- when you wash dishes
- when you pick up the phone
- when you shave
- while riding in the car

Now plan the activities with which you will do your exercises.

Lying session: _____

Standing session: _____

Sitting session: _____

Combining exercises with daily activities is an important step to assure that you will continue to exercise. Continue to use the techniques you have learned to prevent accidents.

Eighth-Week Exercise Calendar

	Day 1	Day 2	Day 3	Day 4	Day 5	Day 6	Day 7
Lying	☐	☐	☐	☐	☐	☐	☐
Standing	☐	☐	☐	☐	☐	☐	☐
Sitting	☐	☐	☐	☐	☐	☐	☐

The Ninth Week

As you gain control over your bladder and experience fewer accidents, your confidence will grow. If you have been wearing protection such as pads or diapers, try to reduce the protection beginning now.

Reducing protection is important because it improves your awareness and your motivation to prevent urine loss. As long as you wear protection, it is easy not to think about using your skills. It makes even the most dedicated person a bit more lazy. Going without protection keeps you alert to the situations and events that cause you to leak urine. It reminds you to use your skills to prevent accidents. It keeps you on your toes.

Furthermore, you will feel freer and more independent in your self-control.

Don't move too fast. If you use an adult diaper or absorbent briefs, begin by switching to a pad or absorbent shield. If you use a pad, go to a thinner or smaller pad or pantyliner. When you are comfortable that you can avoid embarrassment at this level, try going without any protection.

Start by going without protection for just an hour at home. Did you succeed? Try two hours. When you are consistently dry without a pad at home, venture out of your home for a short while without a pad. As you sharpen your skills and master more of the situations and events that cause you to leak urine, stop wearing protection in those situations. Eventually, you may be prepared to eliminate padding completely. Whether you achieve this last step or not, be sure to challenge yourself. Every little bit will help to improve your control.

If you have been keeping a bottle, can, or urinal next to your chair or bed, get rid of it as soon as you feel yourself improving. As the easy way out, it only weakens your efforts to maintain control.

Ninth-Week Exercise Calendar

	Day 1	Day 2	Day 3	Day 4	Day 5	Day 6	Day 7
Lying	☐	☐	☐	☐	☐	☐	☐
Standing	☐	☐	☐	☐	☐	☐	☐
Sitting	☐	☐	☐	☐	☐	☐	☐

The Tenth Week

During the tenth week, you will keep your final-week bladder diary (use the Final-Week Bladder Diary found on the pages that follow). Continue your pelvic floor muscle exercises every day, and continue using the techniques to prevent urine loss while you keep the diary. (You may want to review "How to Keep Your Bladder Diary" on page 14 in Step One.) After you have completed your final-week bladder diary, proceed to Step Five.

Final-Week Bladder Diary　　Day #1　　date: _____

In the first column, write the time whenever you void in the toilet.
In the second and third columns, write the time whenever you have an
　　accident.
For every accident, write the reason in the fourth column.

Urinated in toilet	Small accident	Large accident	Reason for accident

Comments: _____

_____

_____

Total number of accidents today: _____

Final-Week Bladder Diary   Day #2   date: _____

In the first column, write the time whenever you void in the toilet.

In the second and third columns, write the time whenever you have an accident.

For every accident, write the reason in the fourth column.

Urinated in toilet	Small accident	Large accident	Reason for accident

Comments: _____

_____

_____

Total number of accidents today: _____

Final-Week Bladder Diary Day #3 date: _____

In the first column, write the time whenever you void in the toilet.
In the second and third columns, write the time whenever you have an
  accident.
For every accident, write the reason in the fourth column.

Urinated in toilet	Small accident	Large accident	Reason for accident

Comments: _____

_____

_____

Total number of accidents today: _____

Final-Week Bladder Diary Day #4 date: _____

In the first column, write the time whenever you void in the toilet.
In the second and third columns, write the time whenever you have an
  accident.
For every accident, write the reason in the fourth column.

Urinated in toilet	Small accident	Large accident	Reason for accident

Comments: _____

_____

_____

Total number of accidents today: _____

n the first column, write the time whenever you void in the toilet.
n the second and third columns, write the time whenever you have an
    accident.
or every accident, write the reason in the fourth column.

Urinated in toilet	Small accident	Large accident	Reason for accident

omments:

_____

_____

_____

Total number of accidents today: _____

Final-Week Bladder Diary   Day #6   date: _____

In the first column, write the time whenever you void in the toilet.
In the second and third columns, write the time whenever you have an
   accident.
For every accident, write the reason in the fourth column.

Urinated in toilet	Small accident	Large accident	Reason for accident

Comments: _____

_____

_____

Total number of accidents today: _____

inal-Week Bladder Diary   Day #7   date: _____

n the first column, write the time whenever you void in the toilet.
n the second and third columns, write the time whenever you have an
    accident.
'or every accident, write the reason in the fourth column.

Urinated in toilet	Small accident	Large accident	Reason for accident

omments: _____

_____

_____

Total number of accidents today: _____

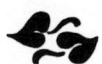

A New Beginning

We will begin our last step together by reviewing your final-week bladder diary, comparing it to your first-week bladder diary, and seeing how much your problem has improved.

Start with the first day of your final-week bladder diary and add up all of your accidents (small and large) for that day. Write that number on the line labeled "total number of accidents today" in the lower right corner of that page. Do the same for each day.

Now, fill in the number for each day here and add them up:

Day #1	_____
Day #2	_____
Day #3	_____
Day #4	_____
Day #5	_____
Day #6	_____
Day #7	_____

Total number
of accidents for
the final week   _____

Next, go back to page 35 in Step Two and copy the total number of accidents from your first-week bladder diary here:

Total number of accidents for the first week   _____

To see how much you have improved, we will compare your total number of accidents for the final week with your total number of accidents for the first week, using the table on figure 15.

First, look down the side of the table and find the number closest to your total number of accidents for the first week. Next, look across the top of the table and find the column closest to your total number of accidents for the final week. Read down that column. Where the first-week line and the final-week column meet, you'll find out how much your problem has improved.

For example, if you had twenty accidents during the first week and six accidents during the final week, look down the side of the table and find the line "20." Then look across the top of the table and find the column "6." Read down the "6" column until it meets the "20" line. The number "70" means that your incontinence has improved by 70 percent.

What Does All This Mean?

If you had no accidents while you kept your final-week bladder diary, your incontinence has improved 100 percent. Clearly, you have every reason to be happy and proud that you no longer have a problem with urinary incontinence. You should continue your pelvic floor muscle exercises every day and keep practicing the strategies you have learned.

You may be tempted to stop exercising your pelvic floor muscles. Don't. You worked hard to strengthen these muscles. If you stop exercising, they will weaken slowly and you are likely to have accidents again. The only way to maintain the strength of your muscles is to keep exercising them. The only way to maintain your new skills for preventing accidents is to keep using them. Incontinence can always return. At the same time, a lifetime of attention to your program may yield a lifetime of control.

If you recorded fewer accidents on your final-week bladder diary, you need to decide whether you wish to pursue an additional method of treatment. Remember, however, that you have been following the program for only ten weeks. If you continue to follow this program every day, you are likely to benefit further over the next four months. We suggest that you give this program a full six months before you decide whether it was helpful to you. At the end of six months, keep another bladder diary, using the Sixth-Month Bladder Diary at the end of this chapter. Then follow the instructions to see how much you improved.

If your problem did not get any better using this behavioral treatment program, you need to ask yourself whether you followed the program closely and paid attention to every detail. If you did not, we suggest that you re-start the program by returning to the beginning of Step Four. If you never got around to going to the doctor, go now.

If you followed the program carefully but you are not pleased with your results, we suggest that you speak to your doctor regarding another method of treatment. Ask your doctor about biofeedback to check whether you have been exercising the right muscles. You may also want to ask about other behavioral training procedures, as well as about medicines and surgery that are appropriate for your type of incontinence.

Total Number of Accidents for

	0	1	2	3	4	5	6	7	8	9	10
90	100	99	98	97	96	94	93	92	91	90	89
85	100	99	98	96	95	94	93	92	91	89	88
80	100	99	98	96	95	94	93	91	90	89	88
75	100	99	97	96	95	93	92	91	89	88	87
70	100	99	97	96	94	93	91	90	89	87	86
65	100	98	97	95	94	92	91	89	88	86	85
60	100	98	97	95	93	92	90	88	87	85	83
55	100	98	96	95	93	91	89	87	85	84	82
50	100	98	96	94	92	90	88	86	84	82	80
48	100	98	96	94	92	90	88	85	83	81	79
46	100	98	96	93	91	89	87	85	83	80	78
44	100	98	95	93	91	89	86	84	82	80	77
42	100	98	95	93	90	88	86	83	81	79	76
40	100	98	95	93	90	88	85	83	80	78	75
38	100	97	95	92	89	87	84	82	79	76	74
36	100	97	94	92	89	86	83	81	78	75	72
34	100	97	94	91	88	85	82	79	76	74	71
32	100	97	94	91	88	84	81	78	75	72	69
30	100	97	93	90	87	83	80	77	73	70	67
28	100	96	93	89	86	82	79	75	71	68	64
27	100	96	93	89	85	81	78	74	70	67	63
26	100	96	92	88	85	81	77	73	69	65	62
25	100	96	92	88	84	80	76	72	68	64	60
24	100	96	92	88	83	79	75	71	67	63	58
23	100	96	91	87	83	78	74	70	65	61	57
22	100	95	91	86	82	77	73	68	64	59	55
21	100	95	90	86	81	76	71	67	62	57	52
20	100	95	90	85	80	75	70	65	60	55	50
19	100	95	89	84	79	74	68	63	58	53	47
18	100	94	89	83	78	72	67	61	56	50	44
17	100	94	88	82	76	71	65	59	53	47	41
16	100	94	88	81	75	69	63	56	50	44	38
15	100	93	87	80	73	67	60	53	47	40	33
14	100	93	86	79	71	64	57	50	43	36	29
13	100	92	85	77	69	62	54	46	38	31	23
12	100	92	83	75	67	58	50	42	33	23	17
11	100	91	82	73	64	55	45	36	27	18	9
10	100	90	80	70	60	50	40	30	20	10	0
9	100	89	78	67	56	44	33	22	11	0	
8	100	88	75	63	50	38	25	13	0		
7	100	86	71	57	43	29	14	0			
6	100	83	67	50	33	17	0				
5	100	80	60	40	20	0					
4	100	75	50	25	0						
3	100	67	33	0							
2	100	50	0								
1	100	0									

Total Number of Accidents for the First Week

the Final Week (or at Six Months)

11	12	13	14	15	16	17	18	19	20	21	22	23
88	87	86	84	83	82	81	80	79	78	77	76	74
87	86	85	84	82	81	80	79	78	76	75	74	73
86	85	84	83	81	80	79	78	76	75	74	73	71
85	84	83	81	80	79	77	76	75	73	72	71	69
84	83	81	80	79	77	76	74	73	71	70	69	67
83	82	80	78	77	75	74	72	71	69	68	66	65
82	80	78	77	75	73	72	70	68	67	65	63	62
80	78	76	75	73	71	69	67	65	64	62	60	58
78	76	74	72	70	68	66	64	62	60	58	56	54
77	75	73	71	69	67	65	63	60	58	56	54	52
76	74	72	70	67	65	63	61	59	57	54	52	50
75	73	70	68	66	64	61	59	57	55	52	50	48
74	71	69	67	64	62	60	57	55	52	50	48	45
73	70	68	65	63	60	58	55	53	50	48	45	43
71	68	66	63	61	58	55	53	50	47	45	42	39
69	67	64	61	58	56	53	50	47	44	42	39	36
68	65	62	59	56	53	50	47	44	41	38	35	32
66	63	59	56	53	50	47	44	41	38	34	31	28
63	60	57	53	50	47	43	40	37	33	30	27	23
61	57	54	50	46	43	39	36	32	29	25	21	18
59	56	52	48	44	41	37	33	30	26	22	19	15
58	54	50	46	42	38	35	31	27	23	19	15	12
56	52	48	44	40	36	32	28	24	20	16	12	8
54	50	46	42	38	33	29	25	21	17	13	8	4
52	48	43	39	35	30	26	22	17	13	9	4	0
50	45	41	36	32	27	23	18	14	9	5	0	
48	43	38	33	29	24	19	14	10	5	0		
45	40	35	30	25	20	15	10	5	0			
42	37	32	26	21	16	11	5	0				
39	33	28	22	17	11	6	0					
35	29	24	18	12	6	0						
31	25	19	13	6	0							
27	20	13	7	0								
21	14	7	0									
15	8	0										
8	0											
0												

Figure 15. How Much You Have Improved

Total Number of Accidents for

Total Number of Accidents for the First Week

	24	25	26	27	28	30	32	34	36	38	40
90	73	72	71	70	69	67	64	62	60	58	56
85	72	71	69	68	67	65	62	60	58	55	53
80	70	69	68	66	65	63	60	58	55	53	50
75	68	67	65	64	63	60	57	55	52	49	47
70	66	64	63	61	60	57	54	51	49	46	43
65	63	62	60	58	57	54	51	48	45	42	38
60	60	58	57	55	53	50	47	43	40	37	33
55	56	55	53	51	49	45	42	38	35	31	27
50	52	50	48	46	44	40	36	32	28	24	20
48	50	48	46	44	42	38	33	29	25	21	17
46	48	46	43	41	39	35	30	26	22	17	13
44	45	43	41	39	36	32	27	23	18	14	9
42	43	40	38	36	33	29	24	19	14	10	5
40	40	38	35	33	30	25	20	15	10	5	0
38	37	34	32	29	26	21	16	11	5	0	
36	33	31	28	25	22	17	11	6	0		
34	29	26	24	21	18	12	6	0			
32	25	22	19	16	13	6	0				
30	20	17	13	10	7	0					
28	14	11	7	4	0						
27	11	7	4	0							
26	8	4	0								
25	4	0									
24	0										

Figure 15. *(continued)*

the Final Week (or at Six Months)

42	44	46	48	50	55	60	65	70	75	80	85	90
53	51	49	47	44	39	33	28	22	17	11	6	0
51	48	46	44	41	35	29	24	18	12	6	0	
48	45	43	40	38	31	25	19	13	6	0		
44	41	39	36	33	27	20	13	7	0			
40	37	34	31	29	21	14	7	0				
35	32	29	26	23	15	8	0					
30	27	23	20	17	8	0						
24	20	16	13	9	0							
16	12	8	4	0								
13	8	4	0									
9	4	0										
5	0											
0												

If All Else Fails

If, after you have exhausted all treatment options available for your type of incontinence, you are still having a problem that interferes with your enjoyment of life, there are other means of controlling the embarrassing and uncomfortable effects of accidents.

For assistance in learning to live with incontinence, we suggest that you read *Managing Incontinence: A Guide to Living with Loss of Bladder Control*, edited by Cheryle B. Gartley. This book describes a number of practical strategies that help incontinent people make the adjustments needed to enjoy an active and productive life. It can be purchased through the Simon Foundation, whose address and phone number can be found on page 113.

There are a number of products and supplies you can buy that will help you live more comfortably with your incontinence, including absorbent pads, external catheters, and compression devices. Help for Incontinent People (HIP) has published a *Resource Guide of Continence Products and Services* to assist people in finding the type of product that would be most helpful for their problem. It can be purchased through Help for Incontinent People, whose address and phone number can be found on page 113.

Absorbent Pads

Absorbent pads may be used to soak up and hold urine. The "adult diaper" market has grown phenomenally over the past several years, and a large variety of products are now available. These products may be disposable, washable, or a combination of both. If your accidents involve small volumes of urine, then menstrual products like pantyliners or maximal absorbency pads may be enough. However, if you leak larger volumes of urine, you may want to use one of the products specifically designed for urinary incontinence. These products are capable of holding large amounts of urine. Some products contain chemicals that decrease odor and increase absorbency. You may also want to use waterproof-backed pads on furniture and bedding.

The "adult diaper" companies continue to improve their products. Most of these companies feature an "800" number in their advertisements. You can call these numbers for information on their latest developments, as well as for assistance in choosing the product that is best for you.

Absorbent products may be purchased at drug stores, supermarkets, or discount department stores. If there is a medical supply house in your area, you may be able to purchase these products in large quantities at a reduced price.

External Catheters

Incontinent men have long used external catheters (also called condom catheters) to collect their urine. The external catheter is a condom that is rolled over the penis. One end of the condom is connected to a tube that drains urine into a collecting bag, which may be fastened to the leg or hooked to the side of a chair or bed. The condom must be changed at least once a day and the penis washed and dried during each condom change to prevent skin breakdown. Long-term use of a condom catheter may cause bladder infection or a urethral diverticulum. Make sure that the condom is not too tight because this may interfere with blood flow and cause damage to the penis.

For women, there are also incontinence collecting bags, which are held in place by an adhesive material, straps, suction, or special undergarments. The bag is connected to a drainage tube that leads to a larger collection bag. Unfortunately, the techniques for fastening the bag around the woman's urethra are less successful than the condom catheter. If you wish to try a collecting bag, you can get information from your pharmacist, your doctor, or the enterostomal therapist at your local hospital.

Compression Devices

Compression devices are used primarily in men. They put direct pressure on the urethra, causing it to remain closed until the device is removed and the bladder is allowed to drain.

The most common device is a penile clamp made of flexible plastic. The clamp is V-shaped when open and, with the penis placed between the "V," the clamp is closed down tightly enough on the penis to stop leakage without causing discomfort.

When pressure devices are used incorrectly, they may cause a urinary tract infection or damage to the penis.

Frequent Urination

Most people use the toilet eight times or less during the day. They void first thing in the morning, every three to four hours throughout the day, and just before bedtime. If you void eight times or less during the day, then you have normal voiding habits. You do not have a problem with frequent urination, and you should skip the rest of this section and proceed to page 113—"A Few Closing Thoughts."

If you void more than eight times a day, you are voiding more frequently than most people. If you feel that this is a problem for you, follow these instructions.

People who have frequent urge feelings tend to void often to relieve the urgency feeling or to prevent accidents by keeping their bladders empty. Do you know the location of every bathroom in town? Do you void every time you get the chance? You shouldn't! Like rushing to the bathroom, frequent voiding can make your problem worse. If you void too often, you are not allowing your bladder to fill to a normal level. If this happens repeatedly, your bladder loses its ability to hold a normal amount of urine. Then your problem with frequent urination or incontinence can get worse.

Further, if you void every time you have an urge, your bladder is still in control. If you want to be in control, then *you* must decide when to void. Don't let your bladder decide. Adopting a voiding schedule and postponing urination is a good method for taking control of your bladder.

Bladder Training: Finding the Right Voiding Schedule

Review the first day of your final-week bladder diary. Look at the first column "urinated in toilet," where you recorded each time you voided. Look at daytime voiding only. How much time passed between voids—thirty minutes? sixty minutes? two hours?

What is the longest time that is comfortable for you? Write that time here:

This is your voiding interval.

Empty your bladder first thing in the morning, every time your voiding interval passes during the day, and just before bed.

Follow your voiding interval consistently during the day. If you have an urge, suppress the urge and wait until your interval passes before voiding. If your time has passed and you don't have an urge, go anyway. Void by the clock, not by the urge. The only exception is when you are about to start an activity that will prevent you from voiding until well after your next scheduled time. If you are going to a show, a wedding, or a dinner, it is reasonable to void just before you leave. That resets your schedule and you should not look for a toilet until after your interval has passed again.

But What Do I Do with the Urge?

If an urge feeling comes on before your voiding interval has passed, use the techniques in Step Four, "Controlling Urge Incontinence," page 77. The only difference is that, after you have successfully suppressed the urge wave, do not go to the bathroom during the first calm period. Instead, get yourself involved in other activities. Take your mind off your bladder until your voiding interval passes, then go to the bathroom and void.

Adhere to your voiding interval until you feel comfortable with it for three days. Only then should you increase your interval by thirty minutes. As soon as you have been comfortable with your new interval for three days, increase that interval by yet another thirty minutes. Continue increasing it by thirty minutes at a time until you are voiding only eight times a day.

For example, if your voiding interval starts at one hour, void when you first get out of bed in the morning. Void every hour during the day, whether you have the urge to void or not. Then, void just before you go to bed at night. When you have been comfortable with this schedule for three days, increase your voiding interval to one and a half hours. Once you have felt comfortable at that interval for three days, increase your voiding interval to two hours. Continue to increase your voiding interval until you are voiding eight times or less during the day.

A Few Closing Thoughts

New and better treatments for urinary incontinence are being studied every day. If you would like further information about incontinence or would like to keep abreast of the newest developments in this area, tell your doctor. Also, there are two nonprofit organizations that serve as national clearinghouses for information about all aspects of incontinence. They are:

Help for Incontinent People (HIP)
P.O. Box 544
Union, South Carolina 29379
1-803-579-7900

The Simon Foundation
P.O. Box 835
Wilmette, Illinois 60091
1-800-23-SIMON

To receive information from these organizations, send a stamped, self-addressed, business-size envelope with your letter.

We've spent a lot of time together lately, and you've worked very hard to help yourself. We hope that you are pleased with your results. We would like to extend our congratulations to you for the success that you have achieved following this program.

We wish you the best.

Sixth-Month Bladder Diary   Day #1   date: _____

In the first column, write the time whenever you void in the toilet.
In the second and third columns, write the time whenever you have an
   accident.
For every accident, write the reason in the fourth column.

Urinated in toilet	Small accident	Large accident	Reason for accident

Comments: _____

_____

_____

Total number of accidents today: _____

Sixth-Month Bladder Diary   Day #2   date: _____

In the first column, write the time whenever you void in the toilet.
In the second and third columns, write the time whenever you have an
accident.
For every accident, write the reason in the fourth column.

Urinated in toilet	Small accident	Large accident	Reason for accident

Comments:
_____
_____
_____

Total number of accidents today: _____

Sixth-Month Bladder Diary   Day #3   date: —————

In the first column, write the time whenever you void in the toilet.
In the second and third columns, write the time whenever you have an
accident.
For every accident, write the reason in the fourth column.

Urinated in toilet	Small accident	Large accident	Reason for accident

Comments: ——————————————————

—————————————————————————

—————————————————————————

Total number of accidents today: ——————

Sixth-Month Bladder Diary   Day #4   date: _____

In the first column, write the time whenever you void in the toilet.
In the second and third columns, write the time whenever you have an
   accident.
For every accident, write the reason in the fourth column.

Urinated in toilet	Small accident	Large accident	Reason for accident

Comments: _____

_____

_____

Total number of accidents today: _____

Sixth-Month Bladder Diary　　Day #5　date: _____

In the first column, write the time whenever you void in the toilet.
In the second and third columns, write the time whenever you have an
　accident.
For every accident, write the reason in the fourth column.

Urinated in toilet	Small accident	Large accident	Reason for accident

Comments:

_____

_____

_____

Total number of accidents today: _____

Sixth-Month Bladder Diary   Day #6   date: _____

In the first column, write the time whenever you void in the toilet.
In the second and third columns, write the time whenever you have an
   accident.
For every accident, write the reason in the fourth column.

Urinated in toilet	Small accident	Large accident	Reason for accident

Comments:

_____

_____

_____

Total number of accidents today: _____

Sixth-Month Bladder Diary   Day #7   date: _____

In the first column, write the time whenever you void in the toilet.
In the second and third columns, write the time whenever you have an accident.
For every accident, write the reason in the fourth column.

Urinated in toilet	Small accident	Large accident	Reason for accident

Comments:
_____
_____
_____

Total number of accidents today: _____

Instructions: How to Interpret Your Sixth-Month Bladder Diary

To see how much your problem has improved after six months of following this behavioral treatment program, review your sixth-month bladder diary and compare it to your first-week bladder diary.

Start with the first day of your sixth-month bladder diary and add up all of your accidents (small and large) for that day. Write that number on the line labeled "total number of accidents today" in the lower right corner of that page. Do the same for each day.

Now, fill in the number for each day here and add them up:

Day #1   _____

Day #2   _____

Day #3   _____

Day #4   _____

Day #5   _____

Day #6   _____

Day #7   _____

_____

Total number
of   accidents
at six months   _____

Next, go back to page 35 in Step Two and copy the total number of accidents from your first-week bladder diary here:

Total number of accidents for the first week   _____

To see how much you have improved, we will compare your total number of accidents at six months with your total number of accidents during the first week, using the table in figure 15.

First, look down the side of the table and find the number closest to your total number of accidents during the first week. Next, look across the top of the table and find the column closest to your total number of accidents at six months. Read down that column. Where the first-week line and the sixth-month column meet, you'll find out how much your problem has improved.

For example, if you had twenty accidents during the first week and six accidents during the week that you kept your sixth-month bladder diary, look down the side of the table and find the line "20." Then, look across the top of the table and find the column "6." Read down the "6" column until it meets the "20" line. The number "70" means that your incontinence has improved by 70 percent.

Now go back to page 102 in Step Five to find out—"What Does All This Mean?"

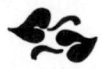

Further Evaluation and Testing

Cystometry

Cystometry (also called cystometrogram, or CMG) measures the pressure in your bladder as it is slowly filled. It allows the doctor to observe how your bladder responds to filling. It takes about thirty minutes to complete and can be performed by any health care professional with experience evaluating urinary incontinence. You will be asked to void immediately before the test.

While you are lying on your back, your genital area is cleaned. A sterile, narrow tube (catheter) is passed through your urethra into your bladder. The catheter is used to fill your bladder with sterile water (carbon dioxide gas may be used instead of water). The catheter is used to measure the pressure in your bladder (sometimes two catheters are inserted into your bladder, one to fill your bladder and the other to measure the pressure in your bladder). An additional catheter with a tiny balloon on the end may be inserted into your rectum to measure the pressure in your abdomen. You will be asked to "hold as much water as possible" because you may feel a strong urge to urinate during the test, especially when your bladder is being filled with water.

First, the doctor measures the pressure in your bladder when it is empty. Then, while your bladder is slowly filling with water, you are asked to indicate when you first feel it filling, so your doctor can record how full your bladder is at that time. Ordinarily, a person begins to feel the bladder filling when it has about five ounces in it. Some people have "oversensitive" bladders and feel full when there is only a small amount of water in the bladder. This suggests urge incontinence. Others cannot feel the bladder filling or feel it only when it is more full. This can be a problem if a person does not realize that the bladder is filling before it begins to empty.

As the bladder fills more, the doctor asks you to indicate when you feel that you must void and then records how much water your bladder can hold and notes whether your bladder is normal or not. The normal bladder is stable; that is, it can hold about thirteen to fifteen ounces of water without contracting. An unstable bladder spasms involuntarily before it reaches a normal capacity. Spasms produce urgency (an intense and often sudden need to urinate), incontinence, or both.

After your bladder is full, the doctor asks you to cough or bear down to see if you lose urine when the pressure in your abdomen increases. If you do lose urine during this part of the procedure, don't be embarrassed. The leakage may be a sign that your problem is stress incontinence.

Finally, you may be asked to void so that your doctor can measure the pressure in your bladder when you urinate. This part of the test may be combined with uroflowmetry (see page 129), in which case it is called a pressure-flow study. A low bladder pressure may suggest a problem with your nervous system causing overflow incontinence.

Cystometry may involve some mild discomfort when

the catheter is put in or removed. If you still have some soreness when you get home, you may find that a warm tub bath is soothing. You may see blood in your urine following the test. If either of these problems persists more than twenty-four hours after the test, call your doctor. Contact your doctor immediately if you experience pain, chills, or fever or are unable to pass urine.

If you have a urinary tract infection, your doctor may prefer not to perform this test. There is a small chance (1 to 2 percent) that cystometry may cause an infection in your bladder.

Cystoscopy

Cystoscopy (also called cystourethroscopy) allows the doctor to examine your urethra and bladder directly. It may be performed at the hospital or in the doctor's office. It takes between ten and thirty minutes to complete and is usually performed by a urologist or a gynecologist. You will be asked to void immediately before the test.

While you are lying on your back with your knees bent, your genital area is cleaned and draped with sterile towels. The doctor passes a narrow, flexible tube, called a cystoscope, through your urethra and into your bladder. The cystoscope allows your doctor to look at your urethra for evidence of blockage or damage to your urethral sphincter. Once the tube is inside, the bladder will be filled with a sterile solution. That allows a look at the bladder for evidence of a tumor, stones, a diverticulum, a fistula, or other abnormalities. The physician can also evaluate the position of your ureters where they enter your bladder. You may feel the need to urinate when your bladder is being filled.

If your problem is urge incontinence, tumors, stones, or a diverticulum may be seen in your bladder. When there is stress incontinence, the status of the urethral sphincter can be evaluated to see how well it closes. When there is overflow incontinence, the reason for urethral blockage may be identified, such as an enlarged prostate or a piece of prostate tissue remaining after surgery in men or a urethral stricture. When leakage of urine is continual, your doctor can look for a structural cause, such as a fistula, an ectopic ureter, or a urethral sphincter that does not close completely. Cystoscopy is also performed to evaluate hematuria, looking for a tumor, polyp, ulcer, or stone that may be causing the bleeding.

Cystoscopy may involve some mild discomfort when the cystoscope is inserted through the urethra, so an ointment may be put into the urethra to numb it first. Occasionally, cystoscopy is performed under general anesthesia, in which case you will need to get special instructions from your doctor regarding the restriction of food and fluid for at least eight hours before the test.

After the test, you may experience burning with urination or frequency. You may see blood in your urine following the test. Report these symptoms to your doctor if they continue for more than twenty-four hours. Contact your doctor immediately if you experience pain, chills, or fever or are unable to pass urine.

Doctors will usually postpone cystoscopy if you have a urinary tract infection. There is a small chance (1 to 2 percent) that cystoscopy may cause an infection in your bladder.

Manometry

Manometry measures the strength of your pelvic floor muscles. It takes about fifteen minutes to complete and can be performed by any health care professional with experience evaluating urinary incontinence.

While you are lying on your back, a small balloon is inserted into your vagina or rectum and then filled with air or water. Then you are asked to contract your pelvic floor muscles. When your pelvic floor muscles contract, they put pressure on the balloon. This pressure is recorded and indicates the strength of your pelvic floor muscles. Weakness of the pelvic floor muscles can contribute to urge or stress incontinence.

There are no special preparations for this test and no risks.

Pelvic Floor Electromyography

Pelvic floor electromyography (EMG, also called sphincter EMG) measures how well your pelvic floor muscles are working. It takes about thirty minutes to complete and can be performed by any health care professional with experience evaluating urinary incontinence.

While you are lying on your back, your genital area is cleaned. Then, one of these methods will be used: A few tiny patches may be placed on the skin near the anal sphincter, inside the vagina, or inside the urethra. A tiny needle or wire may be used instead. A small probe may be inserted into your vagina or rectum. A catheter may be inserted into your urethra. Recordings of the electrical activity of these muscles at rest are obtained. You may also be asked to contract these muscles so that a second set of recordings can be made. Abnormal electrical activity in these muscles suggests a problem with your muscles or nervous system.

There may be some mild discomfort if a needle or wire is used. If you're sore after the procedure, you may apply warm compresses to the area.

People taking blood thinners should ask their doctors for special instructions regarding their medications before the test. If you have a bleeding disorder, your doctor may prefer not to perform this test on you.

Urethral Pressure Profilometry

Urethral pressure profilometry (also called urethral pressure profile) measures the pressure in your urethra and compares it with the pressure in your bladder. This test takes about twenty minutes to complete and can be performed by any health care professional with experience in diagnosing urinary incontinence.

While you are lying on your back, your genital area is cleaned. A sterile, narrow tube (catheter) is passed through the urethra into the bladder, and the bladder is filled with about three ounces of sterile water. The pressure in the bladder is measured. Sometimes two catheters are inserted into your bladder, one to fill your bladder and the other to measure the pressure in your bladder. Then the catheter is slowly pulled back through your urethra, measuring the pressure in various places along the urethra. For you to stay dry, the pressure in your urethra must be greater than the pressure in your bladder. If pressures in your urethra are found to be low, this indicates that the urethra is not closing tightly enough. The urethra may be unable to hold back urine, suggesting stress incontinence. The test may be repeated as you cough or bear down.

Urethral pressure profilometry may involve some mild discomfort when the catheter is put in or removed. After the procedure, you may experience burning with urination or frequency. You may see blood in your urine after this test. Notify your doctor if these symptoms persist for more than twenty-four hours. Contact your doctor immediately if you experience pain, chills, or fever or are unable to pass urine.

If you have a urinary tract infection, your doctor may prefer not to perform this test. There is a small chance (1 to 2 percent) that this test may cause an infection in your bladder.

Uroflowmetry

Uroflowmetry (also called uroflow pattern, urine flow-metry, and free-flow analysis) is a simple test that measures how rapidly you are able to empty your bladder. It takes only several minutes to complete and can be performed by any health care professional with experience evaluating urinary incontinence. It is performed while your bladder is full.

You are asked to sit on a commode and void as you usually would. Under the commode is a special collecting device with a timer on it. It measures how long it takes you to start your stream of urine, the amount of urine that you void each second, the strength and smoothness of your stream, and any dripping after voiding. If any of these measurements is abnormal, your bladder may not be contracting strongly enough or your urethra may be blocked. These are both causes of overflow incontinence.

Because this test requires only that you void as you usually would, there are no special instructions or risks involved.

Voiding Cystourethrography

Voiding cystourethrography (also called voiding cystourethrogram, VCU, or VCUG) is an X-ray examination of the bladder and urethra. It takes about forty-five minutes to complete and is usually performed by a radiologist. You will be asked to void immediately before the test.

First, an X-ray film of your abdomen and pelvis is taken to look at the position of your kidneys, ureters, and bladder, as well as to look for abnormalities of your spine and for evidence of masses, fecal impaction, or kidney stones.

While you are lying on your back, your genital area is cleaned. Then, a sterile, narrow tube (catheter) is passed through your urethra into your bladder and your bladder is filled with a special liquid (contrast agent) that can be seen on the X-ray film. You may experience a feeling of fullness or the urge to void when your bladder is filling. Once your bladder is full, a number of X-ray films are taken from different angles to look at the shape and position of your bladder. A very large bladder suggests overflow incontinence. A very small bladder suggests urge incontinence. A sagging bladder (cystocele) suggests relaxation of the pelvic floor. If the liquid enters your urethra, this suggests a weak urethral sphincter. In women, if the contrast material enters the vagina, this suggests a fistula.

Next, while your bladder is still full, you are asked to bear down. Bearing down may cause your bladder to sag. It may also cause you to leak if your urethral sphincter is weak, suggesting stress incontinence.

Finally, you are asked to void and X-ray films of your urethra are taken to look for stricture or narrowing from prostate enlargement (in men), either of which would indicate blockage. After you are done voiding, one last X-ray film is taken to see whether any liquid is still left in your bladder, suggesting incomplete empty-ing or a diverticulum.

The insertion and removal of the catheter may cause some mild discomfort, and after the test you may ex-perience burning with urination or frequency. You may see blood in your urine after the test. Report this to your doctor if it lasts more than twenty-four hours. You should take fluids freely, unless you have some other medical condition for which you must restrict fluids. Contact your doctor immediately if you experience pain, chills, or fever or are unable to pass urine.

If you have a urinary tract infection, your doctor may prefer to postpone this test. There is a small chance (1 to 2 percent) that this test may cause an infection in your bladder. Also, the test exposes you to some X-ray radiation. The amount of radiation is small and it is not a risk—unless you are pregnant. Therefore, if you are a woman of childbearing age, you should not have this test unless you are absolutely certain that you are not pregnant.

If you have an allergy or sensitivity to iodine or shell-fish, inform your doctor. He may prefer not to perform this test on you.

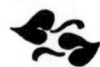

Treatments That You May Be Offered

Behavioral Training Procedures

Behavioral training procedures are a group of therapies that improve bladder control by changing the incontinent person's behavior or environment. Many of these procedures involve learning new skills and strategies to prevent the loss of urine. If you decide to try a behavioral training procedure, you should be prepared to participate actively in your own treatment by practicing new skills and making some changes in your daily routine.

Habit Training and Bladder Training

Habit training and bladder training are methods that alter your voiding habits. They are particularly useful in treating urge incontinence, but they may also improve stress incontinence.

In habit training, you learn your bladder's limits and how to urinate at the right times to avoid accidents. For example, if you know that you have an accident every two and a half hours, you would then void every two hours whether or not you felt the need to urinate.

In bladder training, also known as bladder retraining or bladder drill, you adopt new voiding habits that increase the length of time you can hold your urine.

Habit training and bladder training are procedures that you can apply by yourself. Bladder training is described on page 110 in Step Five.

Pelvic Floor Muscle Exercises

Pelvic floor muscle exercises have been widely used to improve bladder control by strengthening and training the muscles that control urination. They are very useful for urge, stress, and mixed incontinence. They are also known as sphincter exercises or Kegel exercises. Pelvic floor muscle exercises require patience and considerable persistence on your part, but they have helped thousands of incontinent individuals. Your doctor can teach you these exercises in the office. A complete program of pelvic floor muscle exercises and strategies for their use is contained in Step Four.

Biofeedback

Biofeedback is a behavioral training procedure that is used for many problems, including incontinence. Biofeedback has three main components.

- A person's bodily response, such as heart rate, blood pressure, skin temperature, or bladder pressure, is measured.

- That measurement is amplified using a special machine.

- The person sees or hears the amplified measurement.

It is difficult to control actions of which we have little or no awareness. Imagine learning to write without seeing what you are writing; you have much less control without visual feedback. Deaf people who learn to speak without being able to hear themselves don't speak as clearly as people who can hear because they lack hearing feedback. It is visual feedback that allows you to keep your car on the road when you are driving. Biofeedback is based on the same principle. You learn from knowing the results of your efforts.

Biofeedback has been used to alter many bodily functions. Given feedback of one's heart rate, for instance, you can learn to speed it up or slow it down. Feedback of blood pressure makes it possible to raise or lower it. Similarly, biofeedback is used to teach people how to control the bladder and the pelvic floor muscles.

Biofeedback for the bladder was first described in 1948. Bladder biofeedback has been used with men and women with urge incontinence. The procedure is similar to doing cystometry, which was described on page 123 in Appendix A. A catheter is passed into the bladder, and the bladder is slowly filled with water. The difference is that, during biofeedback, you watch the recording of the pressure in your bladder as it is being filled. This way you can see what your bladder is doing. When you can see what your bladder is doing, you are more likely to be able to control it. Watching bladder pressure, you can see when your bladder is beginning to contract. With this feedback, many people can learn to relax the bladder and keep it relaxed long enough to allow them to reach a toilet.

You may experience some mild discomfort when the catheter is put in or removed. There is a small (1 to 2 percent) risk of infection with bladder catheterization.

Biofeedback can also help you learn how to strengthen and control the pelvic floor muscles. Ways of measuring pelvic floor muscle activity are described in Appendix A, "Manometry" and "Pelvic Floor Electromyography," starting on page 127. These tests can be used to provide feedback by measuring the electrical activity of or the pressure created by squeezing the muscles near the urethra, the vagina, or the anal opening. The common thread among these methods is that the action of the pelvic floor muscles is measured and displayed in some fashion for you to see or hear. This enables you to observe muscle activity while learning to contract and relax the muscles at will. After learning to use the pelvic floor muscles properly, many people can prevent stress incontinence by contracting these muscles before and during activities (such as coughing or sneezing) that cause urine loss. It is also believed that contracting pelvic floor muscles can help keep the bladder relaxed. Even when the bladder contracts, accidents can be prevented by tightly contracting pelvic floor muscles.

More than 80 percent of the people treated for urge, stress, or mixed incontinence are improved or completely continent after behavioral training with biofeedback.

Many people can learn to control the pelvic floor muscles without biofeedback. You can start by using the instructions in Step Four. If the instructions that we provide do not help you, it is possible that, despite your careful efforts, you are using the wrong muscles. You may want to consider asking for biofeedback to assure that you are exercising and controlling your muscles properly.

Electrical Stimulation

Electrical stimulation is a method used to contract the pelvic floor muscles artificially. It can be used when pelvic floor muscles cannot be controlled voluntarily. When electrical stimulation was first used for urinary incontinence in 1963, the devices were surgically implanted in a person's body. Today, most stimulators are not implanted. They are small devices that fit into the anus or the vagina. Ordinarily, the devices are turned on for one to two hours at a time, two to three times a day, to keep the pelvic floor muscles contracted.

Encouraging results have been reported with the use of electrical stimulation for stress incontinence and urge incontinence, including incontinence after prostate surgery. People who use an electrical stimulator need to be followed closely by their doctors to assure that it is being used properly and that there are no damaging effects. Although it is uncommon, incorrect use may damage some of the tissues inside the rectum or vagina.

Although electrical stimulation may not be considered a behavioral training procedure in itself, combining this treatment with voluntary exercises of the pelvic floor muscles has been useful, especially if the muscles are very weak.

Medications

Urinary incontinence is often treated with drugs that affect the bladder or the urethral sphincter. Such drug treatment can reduce urge incontinence, stress incontinence, mixed incontinence, and overflow incontinence. If you decide to try a treatment with medications, you must be prepared to take the medicine exactly as it is prescribed by your doctor.

Most medications have side-effects. Usually, the side-effects are minor or short-lived and can be managed by simple measures. However, some people find that they must stop taking these medications because the side-effects make them uncomfortable.

If you have a side-effect while taking one of these medications, don't give up. Tell your doctor about it. It is often possible to reduce or eliminate side-effects by adjusting the dose of the medication. In addition, your doctor may be able to treat the side-effect or recommend simple ways that you can relieve or cope with side-effects. Sometimes, finding the right dosage and adjusting to side-effects can take a little time. If you have decided to try medication for urinary incontinence, be prepared to work with your doctor to achieve the best result possible with a minimum of side-effects.

Because some drugs have effects on unborn and newborn infants, drugs should be taken by pregnant women or nursing mothers only with the consent of their doctors. So, too, if you are of childbearing age, you must be alert to the possibility of becoming pregnant while taking medications.

Urge Incontinence

If you have urge incontinence, your bladder is contracting when it should not. There are several drugs that improve bladder control by keeping the bladder relaxed. By preventing the bladder from contracting, these drugs reduce the feeling of urgency and reduce urine loss. Drugs that are commonly prescribed for urge incontinence include

generic name	trade name
dicyclomine	Bentyl®
flavoxate	Urispas®
imipramine	Tofranil®

| oxybutynin | Ditropan® |
| propantheline | Pro-Banthine® |

Some people who take these medicines complain of having a dry mouth, constipation, or blurred vision. These drugs can also cause dizziness, confusion, heartburn, and rapid heart beat. If the bladder relaxes too much, these drugs can cause retention of urine (the inability to void). Imipramine (which, in addition to relaxing the bladder, tightens the urethral sphincter) can also lower your blood pressure when you stand up. Because these drugs can increase the pressure in the eye, they should be used cautiously in people with glaucoma. Most studies have reported that these drugs help more than half of the people who take them.

In most cases, treatment is started with a single medicine from this group of bladder relaxants. Your doctor adjusts the dosage of that drug to maximize the benefit to you. If your incontinence is cured and you experience no or mild side-effects, that drug may be continued indefinitely. If not, your doctor may adjust the amount of drug that you are taking or perhaps recommend a different medication.

An additional medicine used to treat urge incontinence in women is estrogen. Estrogen is a natural hormone made mainly by a woman's ovaries. It controls the reproductive system and also helps to maintain the tissues of the vaginal area and urethra. As women pass through menopause, they gradually produce less estrogen. If a woman has a hysterectomy and her ovaries are also removed, then her estrogen level drops rapidly. This loss of estrogen can cause the walls of the vagina and urethra to become thin and irritated, leading to a feeling of urgency, frequent urination, and urge incontinence in some women.

Urge incontinence, frequent urination, and the feeling of urgency in postmenopausal women can generally be improved by replacing estrogen. Estrogen can be taken by mouth, in cream form inserted into the vagina, or by an estrogen patch placed on the skin. Estrogen should be used to treat incontinence only in women who are postmenopausal.

In the past, doctors didn't like to prescribe estrogen because they were concerned that it caused cancer. We now know that, when properly used, estrogen is a safe medicine—especially in the low dosage used to treat incontinence. In addition, estrogen is now known to be helpful for other conditions related to menopause, such as the loss of bone strength (osteoporosis).

Some women who take estrogen experience bloating or breast tenderness. Estrogen can also increase the risk of developing gallstones. Women who have had or now have breast cancer or cancer of the lining of the uterus should not take estrogen.

If you have had your uterus removed, estrogen may be given alone. If you have not had your uterus removed, estrogen will be given together with a second hormone called progesterone. This will cause you to have a small amount of harmless vaginal bleeding once a month. The bleeding generally does not cause cramps.

Stress Incontinence

If you have stress incontinence, your urethral sphincter does not stay closed tightly enough, especially when the pressure in your abdomen increases and presses on your bladder. Drugs that contract the muscles of the pelvic floor that make up the urethral sphincter can strengthen the sphincter and prevent stress incontinence. Drugs that are used to strengthen the urethral sphincter include

generic name	trade name
imipramine	Tofranil®
phenylpropanolamine	Ornade® and many other trade names
pseudoephedrine	many different trade names

Some of these drugs are contained in over-the-counter cold preparations. These drugs can cause an increase in blood pressure, rapid heart beat, headache, or dry mouth. They should be taken with caution by people with hyperthyroidism (overactive thyroid gland). Imipramine (which, in addition to tightening the urethral sphincter, relaxes the bladder) can also lower your blood pressure when you stand up.

Estrogen may also be used to treat stress incontinence because it is believed that estrogen helps to maintain the strength and tone of the pelvic floor muscles. When estrogen is lost, these tissues provide less support for the bladder and the urethra.

When treating stress incontinence with medications, a single drug that increases urethral sphincter strength is used for men and premenopausal women. In postmenopausal women, both a drug to strengthen the urethral sphincter and estrogen may be used together. (Estrogen was discussed in detail in the previous section, starting on page 139.)

Mixed Incontinence

Mixed incontinence has elements of both urge and stress incontinence. The problem is twofold: a bladder that contracts when it shouldn't and a urethral sphincter that is too weak to prevent accidents. For mixed incontinence, a drug from the bladder-relaxant group and a drug from the urethral sphincter strengthening group are used together (or imipramine may be used alone, as it does both jobs). In addition, estrogen is usually added for postmenopausal women with mixed incontinence.

Overflow Incontinence

Overflow incontinence caused by a bladder that does not contract properly can be treated with drugs that stimulate the bladder to contract better. In some people, bethanechol (Urecholine® or Duvoid®) increases bladder tone enough to permit the bladder to contract and empty. The effectiveness of this treatment is not completely proven, and the drug can cause low heart rate and low blood pressure.

When overflow incontinence is caused by blockage of the urethra from an enlarged prostate, the drug prazosin (Minipress®) can be useful. This drug relaxes the muscles that surround the urethra and prostate. Relaxing the urethral sphincter may reduce the blockage enough so that urine will flow out. However, drug therapy does not substitute for prostate surgery, if needed. Prazosin can cause your blood pressure to drop, especially the first time that you take it, so you must follow your doctor's instructions closely. This drug may also cause headache, tiredness, dizziness, rapid heart beat, and upset stomach.

Surgery

For some types of urinary incontinence, surgery is the best and only appropriate treatment. For example, when an obstruction or blockage of the urethra prevents the bladder from emptying adequately, surgery is usually necessary. Urinary blockage cannot be left untreated. In addition to urethral obstruction, there are a number of other conditions for which a surgical procedure is the only or the best treatment, such as bladder tumors, stones, a diverticulum, bladder fistula, and ectopic ureter.

If you are considering a surgical procedure, you will need to balance the benefit of the operation against the risk. The benefit is the chance that your incontinence will improve as a result of the operation. The risk is related to the type of operation that is planned, the type of anesthesia that is used, and your general medical condition at the time of surgery. You should have a detailed discussion with your doctor about the procedure to be performed and its success rate, the type of anesthesia that will be used, the past experience of your surgeon with that procedure, and whether your general health is good enough to allow you to undergo that procedure with the smallest risk.

We discuss only the most commonly performed operations for men and women with incontinence. There are many less frequently performed operations. If your doctor suggests one of these less frequently performed procedures, be certain that you understand exactly what will be done, why that particular procedure has been chosen, how many times your surgeon has performed that procedure, and what that surgeon's success rate is—in addition to asking the other questions regarding your risk.

Surgical Procedures for Men with Incontinence

The most common source of obstruction in men is the prostate. It is common for the prostate to enlarge as men reach their middle and older years. Enlargement of the prostate can be due to cancer of the prostate, but more commonly it is due to benign (noncancerous) growth, which is called benign prostatic hypertrophy or hyperplasia (BPH). It is possible for the prostate to grow quite large without interfering with bladder emptying. However, because the prostate surrounds the urethra, it can easily block the urethra as it enlarges, causing difficulty with urination, incontinence, or a complete inability to void (retention).

The most common operation for benign prostatic hypertrophy or hyperplasia is called a transurethral resection of the prostate (TURP). In this procedure, a urologist inserts an instrument, called a resectoscope, through the penis and carefully shaves away the unwanted tissue that is causing the blockage. Most of the prostate remains. If the prostate is too large or if there are other complications, the prostate may be removed through an incision in the abdomen. This procedure is called an open prostatectomy. If there is cancer in the prostate, a radical prostatectomy may be performed. In a radical prostatectomy, the entire prostate and some of the surrounding tissues are removed, usually through an incision in the abdomen.

Prostate obstruction can cause both urge and overflow incontinence. In cases of urge incontinence and blockage of the urethra because of an enlarged prostate, surgery will cure the incontinence in 50 to 90 percent. If a man has urge incontinence, blockage of the urethra by an enlarged prostate, and some disease of the nervous system (such as a stroke, brain tumor, Parkinson's disease, multiple sclerosis, or a spinal cord injury or disease), the success rate is only 50 percent. Overflow incontinence from blockage of the urethra by an enlarged prostate can be cured by surgery in 95 percent of men.

Incontinence after prostate surgery occurs in up to 10 percent of men, usually in those who were incontinent before the operation, who have a disease of the nervous system, or who have had previous operations on their rectum. Incontinence is more likely to occur after an open or radical prostatectomy and is rarely seen after a transurethral resection of the prostate. If incontinence develops or persists after prostate surgery, a man should wait six to twelve months before having a second operation, as the incontinence may get better on its own during the first year after prostate surgery.

A small percentage of men will lose the ability to have an erection after prostate surgery. This happens most frequently after a radical prostatectomy and least frequently after a transurethral resection of the prostate.

More frequently after prostate surgery, a man may note that—although his orgasm feels the same—the ejaculate (semen) flows backward into the bladder instead of out through his penis. This is known as a "dry climax" or "retrograde ejaculation" and is not harmful in any way.

Overflow incontinence after prostate surgery may be caused by a urethral stricture or too much remaining prostate tissue. Both of these conditions require a second surgical procedure.

Stress or total incontinence after a prostatectomy is usually due to damage to the urethral sphincter so that it no longer closes tightly enough to prevent the leakage of urine. Surgical placement of an inflatable artificial sphincter can cure such incontinence in 70 to 90 percent of men. The inflatable artificial sphincter consists of a circular cuff that is placed around the upper urethra, a fluid reservoir that is placed in the abdominal wall, and a bulb that is placed in the scrotum. The cuff, reservoir, and bulb are connected by tubing. The cuff is full of liquid and presses on the urethra, keeping it closed. When the man wants to empty his bladder, he presses the bulb in his scrotum, and the fluid moves from the cuff to the reservoir. While the cuff is empty, it no longer presses on the urethra and urine can flow through the urethra. After several minutes, the fluid automatically goes back from the reservoir to the cuff and the urethra is once again closed.

Sometimes the device does not work properly, it may need an adjustment, or it may cause infection. In these cases, another operation may be needed. When there are no complications and the device works properly, an inflatable artificial sphincter provides a safe and reliable mechanism for controlling urination.

Another treatment for stress or total incontinence is periurethral injection, a procedure that has been used for over two decades. Various substances have been used, but most reports involve the injection of polytetrafluoroethylene (Teflon®) into the tissues surrounding the urethra. This helps to close the urethra by adding bulk. Good to excellent results are seen in 75 percent of cases (85 percent after a transurethral resection of the prostate, 80 percent after open prostatectomy, and 48 percent after radical prostatectomy).

Surgical Procedures for Women with Incontinence

The most common surgical procedures performed in women are done for stress incontinence. Surgery for stress incontinence is an elective procedure. This means that surgery is optional. You will not hurt yourself by refusing surgery, except that you will probably continue to leak urine.

There are a number of surgical procedures for stress incontinence. All of the different procedures have a common goal: to lift the urethra into a better position in the pelvis where it can be adequately closed off during a cough, sneeze, or other activity that causes a sudden rise in pressure in the abdomen.

The Kelly procedure is performed by a gynecologist through an incision made in the vagina. The Marshall-Marchetti-Krantz procedure is performed by a gynecologist or a urologist through an incision made in the abdomen. The Stamey procedure is usually performed by a urologist through small incisions in the abdomen and, at the same time, through an incision in the vagina. Many of the other procedures for stress incontinence are modifications of one of these three basic operations. The cure rates vary from 50 to 95 percent.

If a woman has stress or total incontinence because the urethral sphincter cannot close tightly enough to prevent the leakage of urine, an inflatable artificial sphincter can be implanted (see page 145), a periurethral injection can be performed (see page 146), or a vaginal sling operation can be done. In a vaginal sling operation, a "hammock" is created under the urethra to support and compress it.

Bladder Catheterization

A bladder catheter is a narrow, flexible tube that is passed through the urethra and into the bladder to drain out urine. A bladder catheter can remain in the bladder for a long period (indwelling bladder catheter), or it can be inserted and removed for each emptying (intermittent bladder catheterization).

Indwelling Bladder Catheter

Indwelling bladder catheters are used for overflow incontinence due to obstruction from either an enlarged prostate or a urethral stricture in a person who is unable or unwilling to have surgery. Indwelling catheters may be used in incontinent people for whom any physical movement is uncomfortable or painful, so that they do not need to move to change wet clothing. Indwelling catheters may also be used in people who have or are at risk of developing pressure sores on their skin (bedsores).

There are two channels within an indwelling catheter, one of which drains urine from the bladder. The other has a balloon at the tip which is inflated once the catheter is inside the bladder to keep it there.

Although indwelling catheters are very effective at keeping a person dry, they may leak or become blocked and then need to be changed. Indwelling bladder catheters may cause urinary tract infections, including infection of the kidneys (pyelonephritis), and kidney or bladder stones.

Suprapubic catheters are indwelling bladder catheters that are inserted into the bladder through the skin on the lower abdomen. They are kept in place by inflating a balloon once the catheter is inside the bladder or by stitching the catheter to the skin. A suprapubic catheter may be used when a catheter cannot be passed through the urethra.

Intermittent Bladder Catheterization

Intermittent bladder catheterization is used for overflow incontinence due to the inability of a bladder to contract (an atonic or acontractile bladder) that has not improved with medications.

The catheter has a single channel to drain urine from the bladder. Every three to six hours, the catheter is passed through the urethra into the bladder. After the bladder is empty, the catheter is removed.

In a hospital or nursing home setting, catheterization can be performed by a doctor or nurse. In the home, catheterization is usually performed by a family member or oneself. The idea of putting a tube into one's own bladder can be intimidating at first, but those who need to learn it are rewarded by acquiring the skills to manage their own bladders. The procedure is more challenging for women than men because the opening of the urethra is more difficult to locate. Nevertheless, even young children have been taught to catheterize themselves every day.

There is a small risk of urinary tract infection when performing intermittent bladder catheterization, and the person must be motivated to perform the procedure several times every day.

We have described each method of treatment individually. Frequently, however, more than one method of treatment is used at the same time. For example, your doctor may recommend behavioral training procedures and a medication for urge incontinence or a medication and surgery for stress incontinence.

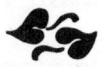

Glossary

acontractile bladder: *see* atonic bladder.

acute incontinence: incontinence that comes on suddenly, usually caused by a new illness or condition and often easily reversed with appropriate treatment of the condition that caused it.

antibiotic: a medication, such as penicillin, used to treat infections caused by bacteria and other microscopic organisms (such as fungi).

anus: the external opening of the rectum.

artificial sphincter: *see* inflatable artificial sphincter.

atonic bladder: a bladder that is not able to contract and empty urine properly, usually because of damage to the nerves that control the bladder. As a result, the bladder fills with urine and remains full, and excess urine that cannot fit in the bladder flows over and dribbles out through the urethra, causing overflow incontinence.

bacteria: microscopic organisms that can cause infection and are usually treated with antibiotics.

behavioral training procedures: a group of therapies that improves bladder control by changing the incontinent person's behavior or environment. *See also* bladder training, biofeedback, habit training, and pelvic floor muscle exercises.

benign: noncancerous.

benign prostatic hyperplasia: *see* benign prostatic hypertrophy.

benign prostatic hypertrophy: noncancerous enlargement of the prostate, common in middle-aged and older men, that may interfere with the flow of urine by blocking the urethra and causing overflow incontinence.

biofeedback: a type of behavioral training procedure that provides visual or auditory feedback of a bodily function, allowing a person to learn to improve control over that function; used to treat urinary incontinence.

bladder: *see* urinary bladder.

bladder catheter: a narrow, flexible, rubber tube inserted through the urethra and into the bladder for the purpose of draining urine or performing diagnostic tests of bladder or urethral function.

bladder catheterization: a procedure in which a catheter is passed through the urethra and into the bladder for the purpose of draining urine or performing diagnostic tests of bladder or urethral function.

bladder diary: a daily record of bladder habits, documenting urination and episodes of incontinence.

bladder drill: *see* bladder training.

bladder fistula: a hole in the wall of the bladder that allows urine to flow out continuously, usually through the vagina in women, and causes total incontinence.

bladder instability: a condition in which the bladder contracts prematurely, which may cause urgency, frequency, and/or urge incontinence.

bladder retraining: *see* bladder training.

bladder-sphincter dyssynergia: the lack of coordination between the bladder and the pelvic floor muscles. Normally, when a person attempts to empty the bladder, the pelvic floor muscles relax, allowing the urethra to open. Then the bladder contracts and urine passes through. With bladder-sphincter dyssynergia, the pelvic floor muscles contract instead, clamping in on the urethra and interfering with the flow of urine.

bladder training: a type of behavioral training procedure that alters voiding habits by gradually increasing the length of time between voids.

bowel: the intestines; the lower part of the gastrointestinal tract.

BPH: *see* benign prostatic hypertrophy.

catheter: *see* bladder catheter.

catheterization: *see* bladder catheterization.

CMG: *see* cystometry.

compression device: device used to put direct pressure on the urethra, causing it to remain closed until the device is removed and the bladder is allowed to drain. *See also* penile clamp.

condom catheter: *see* external catheter.

constipation: a condition in which bowel movements are infrequent and may be accompanied by difficulty passing stool. Severe constipation can contribute to urinary incontinence. *See also* fecal impaction.

continence: *see* urinary continence.

cystitis: irritation or inflammation of the bladder, often caused by infection.

cystocele: bulging of the bladder into the space usually occupied by the vagina, suggesting weakness of the pelvic floor.

cystometrogram: *see* cystometry.

cystometry: a diagnostic test that measures pressure in the urinary bladder as it is slowly being filled to see how the bladder responds to filling.

cystoscopy: a diagnostic test that allows direct examination of the urethra and bladder through a tube (cystoscope) inserted through the urethra and into the bladder.

cystourethrography: *see* voiding cystourethrography.

cystourethroscopy: *see* cystoscopy.

dementia: general mental deterioration affecting memory, emotions, and learning; may contribute to functional incontinence.

detrusor hyperreflexia: *see* bladder instability.

detrusor instability: *see* bladder instability.

dilatation: *see* urethral dilatation.

diverticulum: a pouch or sac opening out from the wall of a hollow organ, such as the bladder.

dyssynergia: *see* bladder-sphincter dyssynergia.

dysuria: pain or burning with voiding.

ectopic ureter: a ureter that enters the bladder too close to the urethra or that enters directly into the urethra or into the vagina in women and may cause incontinence.

electrical stimulation: a procedure in which the pelvic floor muscles are contracted artificially using electrical impulses directed into the muscles; used to treat urge or stress incontinence.

electromyography: *see* pelvic floor electromyography.

EMG: *see* pelvic floor electromyography.

estrogen: a hormone, produced primarily by the ovaries, that regulates the reproductive system and is also believed to maintain the strength and tone of the pelvic floor.

external catheter: a device that surrounds the urethral opening and collects urine.

fecal impaction: a mass of stool that remains packed in the lower bowel rather than being passed normally, which can contribute to incontinence by irritating the urethra (causing urge incontinence) or by blocking the urethra (causing overflow incontinence).

fistula: *see* bladder fistula.

free-flow analysis: *see* uroflowmetry.

frequency: frequent voiding of small amounts of urine.

frequent urination: voiding more than eight times a day.

functional incontinence: incontinence that results from an inability or unwillingness to use the toilet appropriately.

geriatrician: a physician who specializes in the treatment of older adults.

gynecologist: a physician who specializes in the reproductive and urinary systems of women.

habit training: a type of behavioral training procedure in which voiding is scheduled at shorter intervals than those at which accidents had previously occurred.

hematuria: blood in the urine.

hesitancy: difficulty getting the stream of urine started.

hysterectomy: surgical removal of the uterus.

incomplete emptying: not emptying the bladder completely during voiding.

incontinence: *see* urinary incontinence.

indwelling bladder catheter: a catheter that remains in the bladder to drain urine continuously, primarily used to manage overflow incontinence due to obstruction that cannot be repaired surgically.

inflatable artificial sphincter: a surgically placed device consisting of a circular cuff that is placed around the upper urethra, a fluid reservoir, and a bulb—all connected by tubing. The cuff is full of liquid and presses on the urethra, keeping it closed. To initiate bladder emptying, a person presses the bulb, moving the fluid from the cuff to the reservoir, thereby relieving the pressure on the urethra and allowing urine to pass through.

intermittent bladder catheterization: a procedure in which a catheter is passed into the bladder every three to six hours to drain urine; used for overflow incontinence or the retention of urine.

irritable bladder: *see* bladder instability.

Kegel exercises: *see* pelvic floor muscle exercises.

Kelly procedure: a surgical procedure performed by a gynecologist to treat stress incontinence in women. Through an incision in the vagina, the urethra is lifted up into a better position in the pelvis, where it can be adequately closed off during any activity that causes a sudden rise in pressure in the abdomen.

kidney: one of two paired organs (the kidneys) that continually filter the blood to separate out waste products, which are combined with excess water to form urine.

manometry: a diagnostic test that measures the strength of the pelvic floor muscles using a balloon inserted into the rectum or the vagina in women.

Marshall-Marchetti-Krantz procedure: a surgical procedure performed by a gynecologist or urologist to treat stress incontinence in women. Through an incision in the abdomen, the urethra is lifted up into a better position in the pelvis, where it can be adequately closed off during any activity that causes a sudden rise in pressure in the abdomen.

menopause: a period in a woman's life when her menstrual periods permanently stop; the "change of life."

mixed incontinence: incontinence with elements of both urge and stress incontinence. *See also* urge incontinence and stress incontinence.

motor instability: *see* bladder instability.

multiple sclerosis: a chronic disease of the nervous system characterized by fluctuating loss of muscular coordination and strength, as well as bladder problems.

neurogenic bladder: an atonic or unstable bladder associated with a neurological condition, such as a stroke or spinal cord injury.

nocturia: voiding at night.

nurse practitioner: a registered nurse with advanced educational preparation and clinical training in a particular area of health care.

obstruction: *see* urethral obstruction.

open prostatectomy: a surgical procedure in which the prostate is removed through an incision in the abdomen.

overflow incontinence: incontinence that occurs when the bladder is unable to empty properly, either because the bladder cannot contract strongly enough or because the urethra is blocked.

Parkinson's disease: a degenerative disease of the nervous system characterized by tremor, rigidity, and bladder problems.

pelvic floor: muscles and tissues connected to the pelvis which support the pelvic organs (the bladder, urethra, bowel, and, in women, the vagina and uterus) and help control urination.

pelvic floor electromyography: a diagnostic test that measures the electrical activity of the pelvic floor muscles.

pelvic floor muscle exercises: a type of behavioral training procedure that consists of a series of exercises to increase the strength and control of the pelvic floor muscles, thereby improving bladder control.

pelvic floor muscles: a group of muscles that make up the pelvic floor, support the pelvic organs (the bladder, urethra, bowel, and, in women, the vagina and uterus), and help control urination.

pelvis: the cup-shaped ring of bones at the lower end of the trunk, containing the pelvic organs (the bladder, urethra, bowel, and, in women, the vagina and uterus).

penile clamp: a flexible, plastic, V-shaped device that can be closed around the penis tightly enough to close the urethra and prevent the leakage of urine.

periurethral injection: a procedure in which a substance, such as Teflon®, is injected into the tissues surrounding the urethra, helping to close the urethra and prevent urine loss by adding bulk.

persistent incontinence: incontinence that develops gradually over time or remains after other illnesses or conditions have been treated.

polyp: a smooth, inward-projecting growth formed from the wall of a hollow organ, such as the bladder.

postmenopausal: referring to the period during a woman's life after menstrual periods have stopped.

postvoid residual: the amount of urine remaining in the bladder after urination. A large postvoid residual indicates that the bladder is not emptying properly, which may cause overflow incontinence.

pressure-flow study: a diagnostic test that measures the pressure in the bladder and how fast urine flows during urination.

progesterone: a hormone, produced by the ovaries, that affects the inner lining of the uterus; used in combination with estrogen in postmenopausal women who have not had a hysterectomy to treat urge or stress incontinence.

prolapse: *see* uterine prolapse.

prostate: a donut-shaped gland in men that surrounds the urethra between the bladder and the pelvic floor and contributes fluid to semen.

prostatectomy: surgical removal of part or all of the prostate.

prostatitis: irritation or inflammation of the prostate.

pyelonephritis: infection of the kidney.

radical prostatectomy: a surgical procedure performed for cancer of the prostate, in which the entire prostate and some of the surrounding tissues are removed, usually through an incision in the lower abdomen.

radiologist: a physician who specializes in the interpretation of X-ray films, such as voiding cystourethrography.

rectocele: bulging of the rectum into the space normally occupied by the vagina, suggesting weakness of the pelvic floor.

rectum: the lowest part of the bowel.

retention: complete inability to empty urine from the bladder; caused by an atonic bladder or obstruction of the urethra.

spastic bladder: *see* bladder instability.

sphincter: a muscle that surrounds an opening in the body (such as the anus or the urethra), which can open or close the opening by relaxing or contracting.

sphincter EMG: *see* pelvic floor electromyography.

sphincter exercises: *see* pelvic floor muscle exercises.

sphincter incompetence: *see* urethral insufficiency.

sphincter insufficiency: *see* urethral insufficiency.

spinal cord: the thick cord of nerve tissue extending

down the spinal canal (backbone) from the brain, which transmits and receives messages between the brain and the rest of the body; necessary for bladder control.

Stamey procedure: a surgical procedure performed by a urologist to treat stress incontinence in women. Through incisions in the abdomen and vagina, the urethra is lifted up into a better position in the pelvis, where it can be adequately closed off during any activity that causes a sudden rise in pressure in the abdomen.

stress incontinence: incontinence that occurs because the urethra cannot close tightly enough to hold back urine during activities that cause increased pressure in the bladder.

stress maneuvers: activities that increase pressure in the bladder, such as coughing or sneezing; a diagnostic test used to demonstrate stress incontinence.

stress test: a diagnostic test used to demonstrate stress incontinence.

stricture: *see* urethral stricture.

stroke: sudden interruption in blood supply to the brain, frequently resulting in weakness or paralysis of the arms or legs and difficulties with speech and bladder control.

suprapubic catheter: an indwelling catheter inserted into the bladder through the lower abdomen.

Teflon® injection: *see* periurethral injection.

total incontinence: incontinence characterized by the complete loss of control and almost continual leakage of urine, usually caused by a bladder fistula, injury to the urethra, or an ectopic ureter.

transurethral resection of the prostate: a surgical procedure in which part of the prostate is removed by putting a tube (resectoscope) through the penis and shaving away the part of the prostate causing obstruction.

TURP: *see* transurethral resection of the prostate.

uninhibited bladder: *see* bladder instability.

unstable bladder: *see* bladder instability.

ureter: one of two paired organs (the ureters) through which urine flows from the kidneys to the bladder.

urethra: a narrow tube through which urine flows from the bladder to the outside of the body; the opening of the urethra is at the end of the penis in men and just above the vaginal opening in women.

urethral dilatation: a procedure in which a metal rod (dilator) is passed through the urethra for the purpose of opening a urethral stricture.

urethral incompetence: *see* urethral insufficiency.

urethral insufficiency: a condition in which the urethra is unable to prevent urine loss during activities that cause increased pressure in the bladder, resulting in stress incontinence.

urethral obstruction: blockage of the urethra causing difficulty with urination; usually caused by an enlarged prostate in men or a stricture.

urethral pressure profile: *see* urethral pressure profilometry.

urethral pressure profilometry: a diagnostic test that measures the pressure in the urethra and compares it to the pressure in the bladder.

urethral stricture: narrowing of the urethra.

urethritis: irritation or inflammation of the urethra.

urge: the sensation from the bladder producing a desire to void.

urge incontinence: incontinence that occurs when a person is aware of the need to void but is unable to hold urine back long enough to reach a toilet;

thought to be caused by premature contractions of the bladder.

urgency: the intense and often sudden need to void.

urinary bladder: the hollow, muscular organ that both stores urine and empties urine from the body.

urinary continence: the ability to control urination.

urinary incontinence: the accidental loss of urine; wetting.

urinary system: the part of the body that produces, stores, and eliminates urine, consisting of the kidneys, ureters, bladder, and urethra.

urinary tract infection (UTI): infection in any part of the urinary system, including the kidneys (pyelonephritis), ureters, bladder (cystitis), or urethra (urethritis).

urinate: to pass urine; to void.

urine: the waste products filtered from the blood and combined with excess water by the kidneys.

urine flowmetry: *see* uroflowmetry.

urodynamic tests: diagnostic tests that measure the function of the bladder, urethra, and/or pelvic floor muscles. *See also* cystometry, manometry, pelvic floor electromyography, pressure-flow study, urethral pressure profilometry, uroflowmetry, and voiding cystourethrography.

uroflowmetry: a diagnostic test that measures how rapidly a person can empty the bladder.

uroflow pattern: *see* uroflowmetry.

urologist: a physician who specializes in the urinary systems of men and women and the reproductive system of men.

uterine prolapse: sagging down of the uterus into the space normally occupied by the vagina, suggesting weakness of the pelvic floor.

vaginitis: irritation or inflammation of the vagina.

VCU: *see* voiding cystourethrography.

VCUG: *see* voiding cystourethrography.

void: to pass urine; to urinate.

voiding cystourethrogram: *see* voiding cystourethrography.

voiding cystourethrography: a diagnostic X-ray test of the bladder and urethra, performed when the bladder is full of liquid, during stress maneuvers, and during and after voiding.

voiding reflex: the reflex in which the bladder indicates to the spinal cord that it is full of urine and the spinal cord then signals the bladder to contract and empty.

Index